SpringerBriefs in Public Health

SpringerBriefs in Public Health present concise summaries of cutting-edge research and practical applications from across the entire field of public health, with contributions from medicine, bioethics, health economics, public policy, biostatistics, and sociology.

The focus of the series is to highlight current topics in public health of interest to a global audience, including health care policy; social determinants of health; health issues in developing countries; new research methods; chronic and infectious disease epidemics; and innovative health interventions.

Featuring compact volumes of 55 to 125 pages, the series covers a range of content from professional to academic. Possible volumes in the series may consist of timely reports of state-of-the art analytical techniques, reports from the field, snapshots of hot and/or emerging topics, literature reviews, and in-depth case studies. Both solicited and unsolicited manuscripts are considered for publication in this series.

Briefs are published as part of Springer's eBook collection, with millions of users worldwide. In addition, Briefs are available for individual print and electronic purchase.

Briefs are characterized by fast, global electronic dissemination, standard publishing contracts, easy-to-use manuscript preparation and formatting guidelines, and expedited production schedules. We aim for publication 8–12 weeks after acceptance.

Fidelia Cascini

Secondary Use of Electronic Health Data

Public Health Perspectives, Use Cases and Challenges

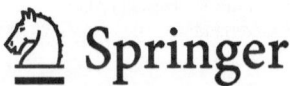 Springer

Fidelia Cascini
Department of Life Sciences and Public Health
Università Cattolica del Sacro Cuore
Rome, Italy

ISSN 2192-3698   ISSN 2192-3701   (electronic)
SpringerBriefs in Public Health
ISBN 978-3-031-88496-2   ISBN 978-3-031-88497-9   (eBook)
https://doi.org/10.1007/978-3-031-88497-9

This Springer imprint is published by the registered company Springer Nature Switzerland AG
The registered company address is: Gewerbestrasse 11, 6330 Cham, Switzerland

If disposing of this product, please recycle the paper.

Preface

I wrote this manuscript by considering those who dedicated their careers to public health to support their functions and activities through a harmonized and discussed collection of scientific developments and best practices reached in the secondary use of health data. I also considered colleagues who believe that improvements in clinical practice, advancements in personalized medicine and the sustainable future of healthcare systems are closely related to the widespread use of data-driven digital technologies, including tools based on artificial intelligence (AI). My thoughts finally have been addressed to sceptics who asked for comparisons of different international experiences and approaches enabling the availability, accessibility, and processing of health data for secondary purposes.

Since the beginning of my career as a medical doctor and fifth generation of qualified doctors in my family, I decided to leave clinical practice focused on single-patient health to pursue an academic and research career in public health. My aim was to work for the safety and success of interventions addressing population health and healthcare improvements because I felt that I could have a greater impact that way, saving more lives. That led me into the areas of legal medicine, health and care systems organization, and governance processes. My major interest has been in complex systems and what strategies, programmes, and plans better support the services delivered for people's health. I have worked extensively in risk management and electronic data research to find solutions to prevent medical errors and unwanted patient outcomes and to optimize healthcare organizational performance and development in clinical research.

During the COVID-19 pandemic, I was engaged by the Italian Presidency of the Council of Ministers as a member of the Emergency Data-Driven Task Force. This experience allowed me to confirm the importance of quickly accessing quality health data to make informed decisions for public health purposes. This experience illustrated the necessity of both finding and accessing e-health data to make intelligent, fact-based decisions on useful methods to manage and recover from such pandemics. My colleagues and I also needed to combine these data from different sources to identify the characteristics of such an outbreak, preventing its evolution and reoccurrence promptly and effectively.

At that time, my collaboration with national and European Union health authorities progressively intensified, becoming very active and pervasive as it is even today. I have worked as a public and digital health expert and adviser embracing the areas of telemedicine, digital vaccination certifications, and technological infrastructures for the primary and secondary use of health data. Consequently, from 2022 to 2024, I was engaged as a national delegate, an expert in the field, to participate in the Working Party on Public Health of the EU Council for the negotiations on the European Health Data Space (EHDS) regulation. I was incredibly satisfied by this position, which gave me the opportunity to contribute to a highly relevant law for the healthcare sector, focused on e-health data use and reuse to bring common and individual benefits while concretely mitigating their risks. To date, by closely working with esteemed colleagues on many initiatives and projects related to the use and reuse of e-health data, including those related to the EHDS framework and its implementation, and further studying how to collect information from the international literature in the field, I have increased my knowledge and strengthened my expertise with the aim of writing an open access book on the secondary use of health data from a public health perspective for all readers, who can take advantage of this approach to inspiring their work.

In this manuscript many different e-health data categories are analysed describing their characteristics and significance, as well as their backgrounds, associated advantages, and risks. With respect to the purposes for secondary use, public interest reasons are mainly related to reporting real-life examples in the fields of epidemiology, health policy making at an international level, clinical research and personalized medicine, patient safety and quality of care, training and developing artificial intelligence tools. Finally, enabling factors and emerging opportunities for increasing health data reuse in public health are presented. These include the digital maturity of healthcare systems through interconnected databases, the frontiers opened by artificial intelligence for health surveillance, disease detection, and resource allocation, the creation of common data spaces sustained by important reforms such as the European Health Data Space Regulation, which aims to standardize electronic health data exchange, empower individuals, and facilitate the reuse of health data by providing precise rules for data governance, interoperability, and safe data sharing across the EU.

These contents are available in the following pages to help the reader visualize and comprehend how to advance understanding of the secondary use of health data, use cases and related challenges from a public health perspective, accelerate interventions aimed at the improvement of people's health and quality of life, advancement and sustainability of health systems, and progress in social and economic conditions of nations.

Rome, Italy   Fidelia Cascini

Acknowledgements

I would really like to thank Ana Pantovic for the constant and dedicated support she gave me during the preparation of the book. I also thank Regina Valenzano and Andriy Melnyk for their significant contributions to edit the final product. I finally thank in advance all the readers who will dedicate their attention to this book to sustain in practice the valorization of e-health data for public health purposes.

Competing Interests The author has no competing interests to declare that are relevant to the content of this manuscript.

Contents

About the Author

Fidelia Cascini, MD, PhD, born in Rome (Italy) on 13 July 1975 and mother of two sons, is a medical doctor specialized in Legal Medicine and Hygiene. She holds a Doctor of Philosophy in Forensic Medicine, a Master of Science in Hospital Risk Management, and is currently professor in the Department of Life Sciences and Public Health at Università Cattolica del Sacro Cuore in Rome.

In cooperation with the Italian Ministry of Health, where she has been in charge since 2021 as digital health adviser, Fidelia has been involved in several European Union initiatives in the framework of the European Health Data Space (EHDS) such as the joint action Xt-EHR (Extended EHR@EU Data Space for Primary Use) and the coordination and support action MyHealth@MyHands (Supporting patients' access to their health data in the context of healthcare services for citizens across the EU) in the field of primary use; the joint actions TEHDAS and TEHDAS2 (Towards the European Health Data Space), and the support actions QUANTUM (Quality, Utility and Maturity Measured) and SHAIPED (Supporting Health Data Access Bodies to establish Artificial Intelligence pathways enabling Deployment of AI as medical device tools), in the field of secondary use of health data.

From June 2022 to March 2024, she has been designated by the Ministry for Foreign Affairs and International Cooperation as the expert, national delegate at the Working Party on Public Health of the EU Council, for the negotiations on the European Health Data Space regulation entering into force in 2025.

In July 2023, she was elected Co-Chair of the Clinical and Consumer Engagement Work Stream at the Global Digital Health Partnership (GDHP) with the main mission of improving the digital health literacy and use of digital health technologies across countries.

In June 2024, she was elected Chair of Stakeholders' Fora within the Health Data Access Bodies (HDAB) Community of Practice for the secondary use of health data in the scope of the European Health Data Space. In February 2025, she has been elected Chair of the Steering Board of the same HDAB Community of Practice.

Since 2024, she is a member of the Advisory Board of the Tendering HADEA/2023/OP/0024 "Capacity Building for Secondary Uses of Health Data for the European Health Data Space".

From 2020 to 2021, she was a member of the G7 Working Group on Standards and Interoperability and the G7 Artificial Intelligence Working Group.

Since 2019, she also has served as Italian Representative of the European Observatory on Health Systems and Policies (WHO).

At a national level, she is currently a member of the National Coordination Centre of Territorial Ethics Committees for clinical trials on medicinal products for human use and medical devices, established at the Italian Medicines Agency (AIFA). She is also the expert of the Coordination Unit of the working group for the creation of the New Portal for Transparency of Health Services at the National Agency of Regional Health Services (Agenas).

From 2020 until the end of 2021, she was a member of the Data Coordination Unit Task Force, established in March 2020 by the Prime Minister's office for the COVID-19 emergency. She acted as digital health expert of the Ministry of Health in the working group on investments for Telemedicine managed by the National Agency of Regional Health Services (Agenas).

In 2021 she was engaged by the World Health Organization (WHO) for "Drawing up a country snapshot on the role of public health agencies and services in responding to the COVID-19 pandemic in Italy" within a global WHO project on how to strengthen public health. She is also a member of the Strategic Partners' Initiative for Data and Digital Health (SPI-DDH) launched in 2024 by the WHO, European Region.

She is currently author of 4 monographs and of more than 70 scientific research papers, of which 57 are indexed on Scopus (almost always appearing as first author) and published in Q1-level journals for research in the field of public health and digital technologies.

List of Tables

Chapter 1
Electronic Health Data Categories

The evolving landscape of healthcare technology has given rise to various types of data, each serving a unique purpose in practice. The definitions of the most commonly used categories of health data are presented in Table 1.1, while the descriptions available throughout the chapter show their diversity and significance, mainly in advancing healthcare research and practice.

1.1 Real-World Data

1.1.1 Real-World Data: Background

Real-world data (RWD) are data related to patient health status and/or the delivery of healthcare and are routinely collected from a variety of sources. Examples of RWD include data derived from electronic health records, medical claims data, data from product or disease registries, and data gathered from other sources (such as digital health technologies) that can inform health status [1]. The NICE further extends the definition of RWD in that most data sources are observational (or non-interventional), meaning that if any interventions (or exposures) are applied, they are not determined by a study protocol but are a result of decisions made by patients and healthcare professionals. Real-world evidence, on the other hand, is evidence generated from the analysis of RWD that provides information about the usage and associated benefits and risks of a medical product [1]. The NICE further elaborates that RWE can include a large variety of evidence types such as disease epidemiology, health service research, or causal estimation. In RWE studies, routinely collected data, customized data collection, or a combination of the two can be used. Single-arm trials that use RWE sources to create an external control are also considered RWE studies [2].

F. Cascini, *Secondary Use of Electronic Health Data*, SpringerBriefs in Public Health, https://doi.org/10.1007/978-3-031-88497-9_1

Table 1.1 Common health data categories

Electronic health data categories	Definition
Real-World Data (RWD) and Real-World Evidence (RWE)—Sect. 1.1	Real-world data (RWD) refer to patient-related health data (namely data representing patient health status and/or the delivery of healthcare) obtained from a variety of sources such as electronic health records, health insurance claims, patient surveys, product and disease registries, e-health services, etc. real-world evidence (RWE) is derived from RWD and represents the clinical evidence about a medical product's safety and risks or benefits
Administrative health data—Sect. 1.2	Synonyms are "health care utilization data", "administrative health care billing records", "administrative claims data", or simply "claims data". These are data that patients generate by encountering the healthcare system, either while visiting the physician's office, undergoing a diagnostic procedure, being admitted to a hospital, or receiving a receipt of a prescription at a community pharmacy. Their collection is primarily intended for administrative or billing purposes; however, they are also used to study healthcare delivery, benefits, harms, and costs
Biobanking data—Sect. 1.3	Data collected in biobanks which represent large collections of biospecimens connected/linked to relevant personal and health information (such as health records, family history, lifestyle, and genetic information) and their main purpose is for use in health and medical research
Clinical trial data—Sect. 1.4	Refers to data collected during a trial including various data types that are later transformed into analysable datasets to answer specific research questions and generate various publications/reports
Electronic Health Records (EHRs)—Sect. 1.5	An electronic health record (EHR) is a digital patient paper chart that contains health information (such as medical and treatment histories of patients) but also medications, treatment plans, immunization dates, allergies, radiology images, and laboratory and test results
Genomic and proteomic data—Sect. 1.6	These data are derived from genomics and proteomic studies. Genomics performs a systematic study of genes, their functions, and their interactions, while proteomics is focused on studying proteins, protein complexes, their localization, their interactions, and posttranslational modifications
National Registries—Sect. 1.7	National health registries represent health information systems, which are primarily intended to collect, process, and analyse data on diagnosed diseases. National registries are usually focused on specific diseases and include only, for example, diabetic or cancer patients, among others
Person-generated (electronic) health data (PGHD)—Sect. 1.8	Person-generated health data (PGHD) includes health-related data that patients (or family members or other caregivers) create, record, or collect, aiming to help address a health concern. This data type often sits outside the traditional clinical setting but can provide useful insights and give a more comprehensive picture of a patient's health. PGHD data sources mainly today include technology-driven solutions such as wearable devices, mobile apps, and home monitoring systems. Such data include results from home glucose/blood pressure monitoring wearable, fitness tracker data, among others
Social and Behavioural determinants of health—Sect. 1.9	Social and behavioural determinants of health (SBDH) include environmental conditions in which people are born, live, learn, work, play, worship, and age that are found to impact a wide range of outcomes and risks related to health, functioning, and quality of life. These variables can be divided into five main categories: Economic stability; education access and quality; social and community context; neighbourhood and built environment; and healthcare access and quality

In recent years, the generation of RWD has grown rapidly as a result of the immersion of new technologies in healthcare sectors in different scenarios. Because RWD is by nature observational, unstructured, or incomplete, and voluminous, it can be viewed as a suboptimal data type that faces both opportunities and challenges. Different research methods are being used and developed to make use of RWD, including clinical trials, target trial emulation, and applications of machine learning (ML) and artificial intelligence (AI) techniques [3]. Organizations such as the Big Data Steering Group (BDSG), the European Medicines Agency (EMA), and the European Medicines Regulatory Network (EMRN) are working to establish a framework that will facilitate the use of and establish values for RWE [4].

1.1.2 Real-World Data: Advantages and Challenges

RWD offers many advantages since it has a wide range of applications, including research (epidemiology, disease burden, and treatment patterns) and the evaluation of the economic value of medical products [5]. The benefits of reusing these data depend on the context and the type of application; however, there are many advantages, the most important of which include the following outlined below.

Enabling time and cost efficiency in new investigations, for example the implementation of RWE in early drug development stages, can decrease both time and expenses in conducting those clinical trials.

Facilitating data collection, as these data are, in many cases, routinely collected either for primary healthcare purposes or, in other stances, are readily available for use.

Enabling longitudinal analyses of large samples, the collection of these data is occurring at a very fast pace and thus generates data that are high in volume and longitudinal in nature.

Providing information and knowledge about outcomes that are otherwise hard to obtain, RWE can complement randomized-controlled trial (RCT) evidence, since these are not sufficient to provide a complete picture of medical products, as adverse events are more routinely tracked in clinical practice [6]. Therefore, regulatory bodies require that manufacturers collect information about safety in the post-marketing period (known as post-marketing studies), which are RWE studies. Thus, when complementing RCT evidence, RWE addresses the gaps in clinical knowledge [7].

- The use of RWD for secondary use in health research poses several challenges that stem from the inherent nature of these observational data. Unlike data collected in controlled settings, RWD is gathered in real-world scenarios, introducing variability and complexity. Moreover, a significant obstacle arises from the unstructured nature of RWD, which encompasses diverse formats such as texts, imaging, and networks. Inconsistencies abound, as data entry is carried out by different healthcare providers and systems, contributing to the messiness of the information.

- The voluminous and dynamic nature of RWDs, characterized by high-frequency collection, further complicates their management and analysis. Incompleteness is another issue, with critical end points often missing, as RWD was originally not intended for analytical purposes. For example, registry data frequently have limited follow-up points, hindering comprehensive analysis. Biases and measurement errors also afflict RWD, exemplified by selection bias in Internet and mobile device data. In essence, RWDs are characterized by their messy, incomplete, and heterogeneous nature and are compounded by various measurement errors and biases.

- It is well recognized that RWD quality is suboptimal and inconsistent [8–11]; as such, assessing and ensuring data quality becomes a challenging endeavour because of the complexity and heterogeneity of the information. Consequently, compromised data quality jeopardizes result validation, reproducibility, and replicability. Despite these challenges, the imperative for establishing best practices in data quality assessment remains crucial, especially considering that the evidence generated from RWD can form the basis for regulatory decisions impacting millions of lives.

- Furthermore, ethical and privacy concerns are inherent in the use of RWD, as the information often includes sensitive details such as medical histories, disease status, and financial information. The risks to privacy are amplified when linking data from different databases, a common practice in RWD analysis. These challenges underscore the need for rigorous ethical considerations and privacy safeguards in the utilization of RWD, as the implications of data analysis extend beyond scientific research to impact individuals and communities [3].

1.1.3   Real-World Data: Examples of Reuse

1.1.3.1   The Use of RWD for Research Purposes

The RWD plays a pivotal role in the secondary use of health data and has been shown to significantly impact clinical research. One notable application is in supporting randomized-controlled trials (RCTs), especially those focused on rare diseases. RCTs face challenges such as methodological issues, high costs, enrolment difficulties, and prolonged durations [12]. To address these challenges, a solution involves implementing a single-arm experimental or synthetic control design, utilizing historical information or data from EHRs and other sources for the control arm. While this study design is not without controversy, it becomes a viable option when investigating diseases with a well-understood course and predictable, fast, and significant treatment effects [13–15]. Additionally, RWE, particularly that obtained from EHR data, informs and optimizes clinical study designs by identifying unmet clinical needs and facilitating the recruitment of cohorts that would benefit the most from new treatments. It also aids in revising study inclusion criteria and identifying suitable study sites, ultimately supporting patient enrolment and retention [7, 13].

Furthermore, RWE facilitates the identification of the most important variables, streamlining data collection to be more costly and time efficient [13]. In the context of patient enrolment, RWE present in registries enhances the recruitment process, which is particularly crucial in rare disease studies where it can be challenging [16]. A notable example is the ADAPTABLE trial, the first large-scale EHR-enabled clinical trial utilizing EHR data to identify and enrol patients [3]. These examples underscore the multifaceted contributions of RWE in enhancing the efficiency and effectiveness of clinical research methodologies [3].

1.1.3.2   The Use of RWD in Clinical and Regulatory Decision-Making Processes

The secondary use of health data has ushered in a transformative era in supporting critical aspects of clinical and regulatory decision-making, particularly in the realm of medical product approvals. Traditionally, the foundation for new drug approvals rested on data derived from traditional RCTs. However, a noteworthy shift has occurred, with RWD now playing an instrumental role in informing decisions related to new drug approvals, supplementary approvals, and label revisions [17]. A compelling illustration of this paradigm shift can be seen in the case of palbociclib, a CDK4/6 inhibitor initially approved exclusively for the treatment of women with ER+/HER2—breast cancer. In 2019, the approval scope broadened to include men, a decision supported by EHR data documenting its off-label use among male patients [18].

1.1.3.3   The Use of RWD in Supporting Regulation Processes

Moreover, RWD serves as a crucial pillar for supporting European Union (EU) regulations. Current pathways for RWE generation for the EMA encompass diverse sources, including EU countries' in-house databases, the Data Analysis and Real-World Interrogation Network (DARWIN EU) [19], and investigations through the agency's research framework contracts. The results from the utilization of these diverse sources of information have proven invaluable in addressing a spectrum of questions and providing support for decision-making processes across various contexts and procedures. This includes addressing the research needs of key committees such as the Pharmacovigilance Risk Assessment Committee (PRAC), Paediatric Committee (PDCO), Committee for Orphan Medicinal Products (COMP), and the Scientific Advice Working Party (SAWP) [4]. RWE contributes significantly in contexts ranging from safety signals and periodic safety update reports to applications for paediatric investigation plans and waivers, maintenance of orphan designations, and scientific advice [4]. This dual application of RWE underscores its versatile and pivotal role in advancing regulatory frameworks and enhancing decision-making processes in healthcare.

1.2 Administrative Health Data

1.2.1 Administrative Databases: Background

The creation of administrative healthcare databases results from the utilization of healthcare services and payments made for payer or hospital billing purposes. These databases are a collection of large amounts of information from thousands or even millions of patients related to their diagnoses, procedures, resource utilization, and costs or charges [20]. These databases are the result of continuing gathering processes, which are often carried out by healthcare providers, healthcare maintenance organizations, health insurance organizations, and other relevant entities such as the civil registry.

Typically, administrative health databases are categorized as "big data", mainly because of certain characteristics of this type of data, including a large volume of information, high speed of data generation, and wide application fields [21].

In general, data gathering in such databases is not explicitly planned for research purposes. Administrative databases focus on preserving financial and administrative details to serve the interests of medical insurers and providers. In contrast, for example, EHRs are predominantly employed by clinicians to record the clinical conditions of patients. This implies key advantages and disadvantages of administrative databases compared with other data sources; for example, owing to the massive amount of data collection, these data allow for large epidemiologic surveys and precise epidemiologic surveillance, but they may suffer from various forms of information bias and a lack of generalizability of the results [22].

1.2.2 Administrative Databases: Advantages and Challenges

Administrative health data have become a powerful research tool for epidemiologists. Owing to its own nature, strengths and limitations are present within this type of data. A summary is presented in Table 1.2.

Current administrative databases still present issues within several types of studies. This can cause a flaw in the analysis resulting from these data or make the collected data inefficient for certain analysis purposes, limiting their secondary use. For example, in the Lombardia region (Italy), abnormal mortality rates were found due to a change in coding status during a study [25]. In general, the use of billing and coding data in research offers large sample sizes and increased statistical power, enabling multivariate adjustments for risk factors. However, potential limitations arise from the data source (i.e. nonbillable clinical events may not be registered), coding issues, linkages between multiple sources, lack of validation, and confounders not available for assessment. Additionally, variations in the definition of diseases across different hospitals or healthcare structures may introduce observer bias, emphasizing the need for careful consideration of these factors in the various applications of data [26].

Table 1.2 Advantages and limitations of administrative databases

Strengths	Limitations
Very large sample size with a diverse population basis	Lack of additional clinical information due to a bias of use for administrative and billing purposes
Large number of variables and good heterogeneity and accessibility	
Enabling faster and less expensive research	Selection bias may be present due to consent requirements, etc.
Patients are followed over extended periods of time	Potential data gaps due to heterogeneous or changing coding practices in the field
More comprehensive dataset when properly linked	Clinical significance of administrative data is not always evident
Easier identification of rare or reduced patient populations, i.e. rare diseases, etc. [23]	Misclassification of data may turn into jeopardized study results [24]

1.2.3 Administrative Databases: Examples of Reuse

1.2.3.1 The Use of Administrative Health Data in Research

In the realm of secondary use of electronic health data, administrative databases offer valuable resources for diverse research endeavours. Population-based epidemiological studies benefit significantly from these databases, enabling the evaluation of crucial indicators such as incidence, prevalence, and temporal trends in specific diseases or health conditions, along with associated mortality rates. For example, a comprehensive epidemiological study on heart failure was conducted, encompassing 2.1 million inhabitants of Sweden, using data collected posthospital admission [27]. Similarly, trends in diabetes incidence, prevalence, and mortality rates over a decade were explored by employing hospital discharge abstracts and physician service claims [28].

1.2.3.2 The Use of Administrative Health Data in Quality-of-Care Studies

Outcome studies provide a platform to research demographic characteristics and major medical conditions over an extended period, offering a representative sample for the general population, as exemplified in a ten-year study on the incidence and short-term outcomes of acute myocardial infarction in the Netherlands [29]. Administrative health data also provide benefits in quality-of-care studies, facilitating the evaluation of healthcare services and systems. Organizations such as the Agency for Healthcare Research and Quality (AHRQ) have introduced quality indicators on the basis of in-hospital discharge abstracts, which serve as tools for highlighting quality concerns and tracking changes over time [30]. Predictive models can contribute to quality-of-care improvement by identifying high-risk patients for targeted interventions, thus reducing hospitalizations [31].

1.2.3.3   The Use of Administrative Health Data in Detecting Adverse Events

Moreover, administrative databases offer a unique opportunity for adverse drug event studies, given their capacity to study large sample sizes over extended observation periods. Although advantageous, challenges arise from the lack of information on covariates and their potential impact on outcomes, as illustrated by the use of ICD-9-CM codes to detect adverse drug reactions (ADRs), which results in a chart with a positive predictive value ranging between 60% and 100% [32]. These examples underscore the versatility of administrative databases in supporting diverse research domains within the secondary use of electronic health data.

1.3   Biobanking Data

1.3.1   Biobanking Data: Background

The Declaration of Taipei defined "a collection of biological materials and associated data" as a biobanking term was first used by Loft and Poulsen [33]. Since then, the application of these data has expanded due to the advancement of omics science and the possibility of utilizing large databases in the health field. The term "biobanking" is often improperly applied to any collection of human biospecimens, without considering the ethical and legal requirements or the standardization of a variety of processes related to tissue collection. Biobanks represent large biospecimen collections that are linked to relevant personal and health information, such as health records, family history, lifestyle, and genetic information, whose primary aim is utilization in medical and health research [34]. This is aligned with the definition provided by the Organisation for Economic Co-operation and Development (OECD), which defines biobanks as organized resources intended for genetic research, encompassing human biological materials, data derived from genetic analysis, and related information [35]. According to the Declaration of Taipei, a biobank is "a collection of biological materials and associated data", whereas a health database is "a system for collecting, organizing and storing health information" [36].

Biobanking plays a primary role in the new era of precision medicine and has enormous potential but also poses potential dangers, especially in terms of data sensitivity. Biobanks also support both public health and patient care efforts by providing resources for scientific and medical research [37, 38]. As biobanking data are ultimately collected from populations and individuals, concerns about crucial aspects related to human rights, such as dignity, autonomy, privacy, confidentiality, and non-discrimination, among others, increase the importance of promoting advancement in the biobanking field while individual rights are protected [39].

1.3.2   Biobanking Data: Advantages and Challenges

In the realm of secondary use of health data, the utilization of biobanking data offers a myriad of advantages. One significant benefit lies in the potential for a larger sample size and greater data diversity, enabling a more comprehensive understanding of various health conditions. Moreover, this trend is likely to continue with the existence of efficient recruitment methods that facilitate ongoing enrolment; for example, the recruitment target of the Kaiser Permanente and Million Veterans Program (MVP) is over 85,000 participants per year [40]. Furthermore, biobanking offers the ability to include a greater degree of race/ethnic diversity than many clinical research studies do, thereby overcoming the bias introduced by restricting studies to a single race/ethnic group. An example of this effort was made by the MVP, which recruited between 15% and 20% of their sample to be of African ancestry [41]. The benefit of merging these two data sources also lies in the fact that by genotyping the participants only once, there is the possibility of defining multiple case groups, which emphasizes the potential for efficient use of biobank data. Furthermore, given that the EHR data are gathered continuously during each repeated healthcare encounter, there are vast longitudinal data that can facilitate longitudinal follow-up studies focusing on incident events, recurrent events, response to treatments, and transitions in health over time [42]. Although the burden of rare diseases is high (e.g. in the United States), rare disease studies are often less supported than those of common diseases. The obstacle also lies in the need to collect large sample sizes for the genetic discovery of rare diseases. Therefore, linking electronic health records (EHRs) with biobanking increases the potential to identify and recruit rare disease cases and their family members, facilitating the conduct of diagnostic and therapeutic clinical studies. Such large-scale efforts have been made in the United States [43] and the UK [44]. Such large cohorts of genotyped individuals also enable the characterization of a sufficient number of rare genetic variants, which also require a large sample size to obtain accurate results [40]. Moreover, compared with traditional prospective cohort studies, which usually ascertain only a narrow range of phenotypes and assess risk factors once at baseline, EHRs linked with biobanks prove to be cost effective for collecting data on all clinically significant outcomes [40]. Finally, linking EHRs with biobanks enhances the opportunities for utilizing genetic data for personalized medicine, since it can both facilitate the discovery of genetic determinants of disease by conducting observational studies and perform genotype-based interventional studies at scale in the same population [40, 45].

However, their advantages come with their set of challenges. One of the challenges in analysing massive amounts of genetic data is combining biobanks around the globe, which are the basis for conducting comprehensive studies and improving the equity of obtaining genetic data in human genome research. Given that they aim to draw conclusions that should enhance population health globally (such as those related to genetic testing, disease diagnosis, and therapeutic solutions), they should not be based on a biased sample [46, 47]. Thus, to achieve this data diversity at the geographical level, there is a need for a collective effort from researchers involved in genetic studies that use biobanks around the world. This goal is emphasized by initiatives such as the H3Africa Consortium [48], GenomeAsia100K Consortium [49], and the work of Robine and Varmus [50]. These initiatives underscore the importance of diverse datasets for producing robust and generalizable results.

Despite their great potential, biobanks are also considered dangerous to human rights since they are a source of sensitive data that can be accessed. In this context, the World Medical Association (WMA) published the Declaration of Taipei, which serves as a guideline for collecting, storing, and using identifiable data and biological material that are not intended only for their primary use [36]. Given that health databases and biobanks contain data from individuals and populations, concerns related to dignity, autonomy, privacy, confidentiality, and discrimination have arisen. This declaration outlines the need for harmonization between scientific advancements and the protection of individuals' rights, especially regarding the data obtained from their biospecimens. This is the first international guideline that addressed ethical issues and provided associated directions related to activities associated with human databanks and biobanks [39].

Since biospecimen data are linked with associated personal health data such as those contained in EHRs, issues associated with data quality are also present, such as data (in)completeness, missing data, inaccurate phenotype classification, and selection bias [51, 52]. Furthermore, there is inherent population bias, since people are either willing or not willing to share their data through biobanks, and those who are willing are more likely to self-report white race, higher educational attainment, and lower religiosity [53].

Appropriate informed consent (IC) is highly discussed as a crucial topic for biobanking data [54]. Despite the fact that the GDPR-2018 provides important indications for informed consent guidelines, at the moment, unfortunately, no international consensus on informed consent has been produced, leading to differences and intense debates in the interpretation and implementation of informed consent practices. To date, most biobanks have adopted a "broad consent model", basically meaning that biobanks have the right to use samples collected within a specified timeframe without the need to contact patients. However, other more ethical formats, such as "dynamic consent", also arise as a result of the possibility of using information technology tools for this purpose [55].

Effective data management is imperative for maximizing the utility of biobanking data. The Findability, Accessibility, Interoperability, and Reusability (FAIR) principles have recently been introduced to address issues of interoperability and data harmonization in biobanks [56]. These principles serve as a framework for ensuring that data are easily discoverable, accessible, and reusable across different research endeavours. Further attempts have been made by different authors to extend the FAIR principles and provide further requirements on data quality, specifically in the field of biobanking [57–59].

The international harmonization of biobanks has been a concerted effort over the past two decades. Many countries have established specific legislation or guidelines for the collection and processing of human tissues [60]. The best practices guidelines for human and microorganism biological resources were published by international entities such as the Organization for Economic Co-operation and Development (OECD) [61], the International Society for Biological and Environmental Repositories (ISBER) [62], the National Cancer Institute (NCI) [63], the International Agency for Research on Cancer (IARC) [64], the Council for International Organizations of Medical Sciences (CIOMS) [65], the Nuffield Council on bioethics [66], and the European Society of Human Genetics [67]. Additionally, many countries have developed legislation and guidelines for human tissue collection and processing at the national and regional levels. Nevertheless, there is a recognized need for internationally harmonized criteria for sample collection, aiming to merge major requirements into a unified global standard for biobanking. This endeavour seeks to standardize information on the collection, access, and research activities in human data and biological resources, fostering collaboration and advancing the secondary use of health data on a global scale. To address this requirement, a working group was organized that comprises more than 70 experts from 29 countries at the ISO Technical Committee "Biotechnologies" and works on an international standard for biobanking (ISO 20387) that was published in 2018; this group relies on 14 national and international guidelines and standards [68]. This overarching standard is applicable to all organizations that are involved in biobanking of human, animal, fungus, and plant specimens, as well as microorganisms for research and development [69].

1.3.3 Biobanking Data: Examples of Reuse

The United Kingdom A prospective cohort study of 500,000 participants aged 40–69 years was produced starting with baseline assessments from 2006 to 2010 with the aim of researching the lifestyle, environmental and genomic determinants of life-threatening and disabling diseases of middle and old age. The data from participants include blood and urine biomarkers, as well as a series of web-based questionnaires and ongoing assessments of multimodal imaging and cardiac monitoring performed on target populations [70]. Participants have now been followed up for over a decade, with more than 52,000 incident cancer cases recorded and over 26,000 researchers worldwide currently using the data, positioning the UK Biobank to transform the understanding of cancer [69].

In the UK, a smaller study performed using data from 4509 tests explored the contributions of demographic, social, health, and other medical and environmental factors to COVID-19 risk [71]. These different examples highlight the potential adaptability and scalability of biobanking data to suit multiple population samples, objectives, etc.

Canada The Statistics Canada Biobank is an integral part of the Canadian Health Measures Survey. It collects and stores information from questionnaires; physical measures; and whole blood, plasma, serum, buffy coat, and DNA from consenting

Canadians between the ages of 3 and 79 years on an ongoing basis. Canadian researchers can apply to the programme to use biospecimens for research purposes [72].

China The China Kadoorie Biobank survey took place from 2004 to 2008 in ten geographically defined regions. Over 500,000 adults aged 30–79 years were recruited for the collection of data (mean blood pressure, body mass index, diabetes status, etc.) as well as blood samples (99.98% of the population). The final population had food reproducibility but large heterogeneity by age, sex, and study area [73]. Currently, this study represents one of the world's largest prospective cohort studies, with resurveys produced in 2008, 2013, and 2020 [74].

Japan The BioBank Japan (BBJ) project was launched in 2003 as a registry of patients diagnosed with any of the 47 common diseases selected for this purpose. Participants were enrolled from 2003 to 2008 and followed up until 2013. A total of 200,000 participants were registered in the study [75]. Since 2018, BBJ has been operated and managed as a project aiming to promote registered data and samples, with more than 500 papers based on BBJ samples and information published at the time [76].

Estonia The Estonian Biobank cohort is a volunteer-based sample of the Estonian resident adult population (>18 years), representing the largest epidemiological cohort of the Baltic region. The resulting database, which was collected through a network of medical professionals from Estonia (1.3 M population), allows for wide epidemiological and genomic research [77]. Currently, it comprises a cohort of more than 200,000 individuals and contains more than 700,000 single-nucleotide polymorphisms (SNPs), the most common type of genetic variation among people [78].

1.4 Clinical Trial Data

1.4.1 Clinical Trial Data: Background

The progress in transitioning from paper-based to electronic health data systems has also led researchers to increasingly consider different types of electronic data, including clinical trial registries, as important tools for investigation. According to the WHO, clinical trials and clinical intervention studies include any study that evaluates the health-related effects of interventions (such as drugs or medicines, cells and other biological products, surgical procedures, radiological procedures, devices, behavioural treatments, changes to the care pathway, preventive care, or other treatments) on human subjects [79]. The US National Institutes of Health (NIH) defines a clinical trial as a research study that prospectively assigns one or more human subjects to one or more interventions (which may consist of placebo or other control) to elucidate their impact on health-related biomedical or behavioural outcomes [80].

Pharmaceutical companies and the research community are encouraged to share their data for secondary purposes and thus accelerate scientific discoveries and informed decision-making practices. Since 2013, international organizations such as the US National Institutes of Health (NIH), the Food and Drug Administration (FDA), and the European Medicines Agency (EMA) have developed policies and recommendations for clinical trial data sharing practices [81–83]. Other organizations have also called for improvements, specifically in terms of increased data sharing, with a focus on those generated by publicly funded research. Organizations such as the Organisation for Economic Co-operation and Development (OECD), the European Commission (EC), and the NIH have advocated that "publicly funded research is a public good produced for public interest", which therefore should translate into a responsible but open sharing of information, including clinical research [84]. The sharing of data from clinical research, therefore, can be justified from multiple grounds, including scientific, economic, ethical, etc. [85]. Furthermore, access to data to improve health is strongly related to the right to health and healthcare access. Institutions such as the Medical Research Council (MRC) have promoted principles that aim to determine principles for better use of clinical trial data in the future. Within these principles, transparency is presented as one of the key pillars to aim for research findings that will be as open, understandable, and reproducible as possible [86]. One way to ensure transparency in conducting clinical trials is prospective registrations of study protocols, which can be found in clinical trial registries, such as ClinicalTrials.gov. These registries represent another relevant and important source of clinical trial data and contain a vast number of metadata, including data characteristics from trials, protocols, funding, scientific leadership, etc. [87].

The European Health Data Space (EHDS) Regulation[1] includes data from clinical trials, clinical studies, and clinical investigations, which are subject to Regulation (EU) 2014/536, Regulation (EU) 2024/1938, Regulation (EU) 2017/745, and Regulation (EU) 2017/746, respectively, among the minimum categories of electronic health data for secondary use (Article 51). According to the EHDS regulation, to protect intellectual property rights or trade secrets (using legal, organizational, and technical measures), these data should be included when the clinical trial or clinical investigation has ended, without affecting any voluntary data sharing by the sponsors of ongoing trials and investigations. The health data access body (HDAB) can assess how to preserve this protection while also enabling access to such data for health data users to the extent possible.

---

[1] https://health.ec.europa.eu/publications/proposal-regulation-european-health-data-space_en

1.4.2   Clinical Trial Data: Advantages and Challenges

Within the realm of the secondary use of health data, clinical trial data have emerged as a valuable resource, highlighting both advantages and challenges. Leveraging existing data stands as a primary advantage, mitigating the need for redundant research efforts and fostering a more efficient use of resources [85, 86]. The ability to utilize larger sample sizes by aggregating data from multiple trials also enhances the statistical power and reliability of the findings. As already mentioned, larger sample sizes can facilitate the study of rare diseases or conditions that may not be adequately represented in individual trials. Furthermore, pooled data can help identify rare adverse effects or long-term safety concerns that single studies might miss. The reuse of clinical trial data enables the aggregation of information for meta-analyses, facilitating the re-examination and validation, or correction, if necessary, of existing results. Compared with conducting original clinical trials, this process not only enhances the validity of the data but also contributes to cost efficiency and time savings. Furthermore, the opportunity to test new hypotheses emerges as a noteworthy advantage in the exploration of clinical trial data [85, 86]. Finally, clinical trial data have been applied in regulatory and policy decisions by supporting regulatory submissions for new indications or approvals of treatments in different populations. It is also used in healthcare policy decision-making, as pharmacoeconomic analyses and comparative effectiveness research based on reused data can inform healthcare policy and reimbursement decisions. Finally, reusing existing clinical trial data can be applied more broadly to different populations, improving public health outcomes [88–90].

However, challenges persist in the secondary use of clinical trial data, necessitating further refinement of current practices. The complexities inherent in trial design and data sharing demand continuous improvement, posing questions about achieving full optimization. Standardization issues across various recording practices in trials create complexities for secondary analysts, potentially hindering a comprehensive understanding of the generated data. Additionally, a significant time investment is required for data to become fully available for analysis, impacting research efficiency and efficacy. Another important barrier to the secondary use of trial data is the lack of clarity around the availability of data. Notably, trial repositories do not provide sufficient descriptions of the trial setting, objectives, and design, whereas data dictionaries and schemas describing the dataset's content are often incomplete [91]. For example, discrepancies were found in reporting death events between trials, with variations in reporting deaths during or after the trial. Such differences may impede the ability to make meaningful comparisons between trials, and the delayed discovery of such information can affect the final interpretation of results [92].

Moreover, challenges specific to ClinicalTrials.gov further complicate the landscape of clinical trial data reuse. Issues such as missing or underspecified data, including outcome measures, study design, and conditions not denoted by Medical Subject Heading (MeSH) terms, pose hurdles for effective information retrieval and utilization [87]. The recognition of these challenges underscores the importance of ongoing efforts to increase the accessibility, standardization, and completeness of clinical trial data for their successful secondary use in advancing medical research and knowledge.

Further complications are posed by the complexity of study designs, and tackling this issue might be challenging, and this is exaggerated even more when pooling and reusing of data is performed from multiple sources. Pooled analyses are prone to biases due to sample heterogeneity since even slight differences between datasets can introduce such problems. Addressing the inherent problem of heterogeneity when pooling data from multiple studies can rely on carefully designed protocols (very similar to those required for original clinical trials), which again need very detailed information from the original studies that are used for data pooling. Another way to address this problem is by encouraging close collaboration between secondary users and primary clinical trialists to prevent misunderstanding of trial complexities and nuances by secondary users [93]; however, this approach is not always easy to implement. Overcoming these complexities is crucial if secondary analysis is considered an important outcome itself, for which case, trial protocols should therefore improve their standards for clinical trial documentation and design with secondary analysis in mind [92].

1.4.3   Clinical Trial Data: Examples of Reuse

Patient-Level Data Were Used to Analyse Standard-of-Care Medications from Eight Prostate Cancer Clinical Trials. Data from eight prostate cancer clinical trials obtained from the Project Data Sphere® portal were analysed, with a total of 4127 subjects being combined, integrated, and studied. Among the participants, different heterogeneous demographic data, as well as different cancer stages, were present. By combining comparator arms from different trials, investigators were able to identify possible adverse survival outcomes for surgical castration therapy in prostate cancer patients [94].

Using an Integrated Clinical Trials Dataset for the Identification of Endophenotypes of Alzheimer's Disease Progression. Longitudinal patient-level data for 1160 Alzheimer's disease patients receiving placebo or no treatment with a follow-up of 18 months were investigated. At least three subgroups of Alzheimer's disease patients were identified by the results "learned" from clinical data, each of which is distinguished by a deterioration in cognitive function [94].

Optimizing Trial Design by Integrating Model-Based Clinical Trial Simulation, Pharmacoeconomics, and Value of Information. For example, whether clinical trial simulations based on a pharmacometric model can be utilized to generate prior distributions of treatment effects for Bayesian trial design when treatment effects estimated from previous studies are not suitable has been investigated. Several steps involved in simulating trial outcomes for different trial designs that can be used to optimize trial design while maximizing the return on investment were identified. A case study of febuxostat versus allopurinol for treating hyperuricaemia in gout patients was performed. Different trial design scenarios vary in terms of alternative treatment doses, inclusion criteria, input uncertainty, and sample size. The optimal trial sample sizes varied depending on the uncertainty of the model inputs, trial inclusion criteria, and treatment doses. This interdisciplinary framework for trial design and sample size calculation can be valuable for supporting decisions in later stages of drug development. It can also help identify costly sources of uncertainty, thereby informing future research and development strategies [95].

Using Clinical Trial Data to Conduct Meta-analyses Revealed That Widely Used Treatments Are Not Effective or Safe. The safety of rosiglitazone (a widely used drug in the treatment of type 2 diabetes mellitus) was investigated through a meta-analysis to determine its impact on unexplored outcomes such as cardiovascular morbidity and mortality. After pooling data from 42 randomized-controlled trials, the study revealed an association between the use of rosiglitazone and an increased risk of myocardial infarction (with an odds ratio (OR) of 1.43, 95% confidence interval [CI], 1.03 to 1.98; $P = 0.03$) and an increased risk of death from cardiovascular causes, although with borderline significance (OR = 1.64, 95% CI, 0.98 to 2.74; $P = 0.06$) [96]. The safety of incorporating immune checkpoint blockade into perioperative cancer therapy as a therapy that has proven to be successful in clinical practice is another result. An association between the addition of immune checkpoint blockade to perioperative therapy and an increase in grade 3–4 treatment-related adverse events and adverse events that lead to treatment discontinuation was observed. These results emphasize the need for close safety monitoring in future clinical trials that assess neoadjuvant or adjuvant immune checkpoint blockade therapy [97].

1.5   Electronic Health Records

1.5.1   Electronic Health Records: Background

EHRs represent electronic records of patient health information generated over time whenever the patient has received health or care services. The information included in these records is patient demographics, progress notes, problems, medications, vital signs, past medical history, immunizations, laboratory data, and radiology reports [98]. In addition to containing primary information, data from other hospital information systems are included in an EHR (e.g. imaging data from the radiology department and genomics data from the genetic department). In addition to containment, EHRs can generate reminders for routine screenings and disease reporting or generate graphical trends against various parameters such as blood pressure and blood glucose level monitoring [99].

Since the incentivization schemes of different governments, including the US government, took place, a high adoption rate of these technologies has taken place in hospitals and health offices, with countries such as the United States experiencing an 80% adoption rate at hospitals, naturally leading to further use of these data for research purposes [100].

Despite this improvement in the digital recording of health data and technology used for this purpose, some factors are still missing, especially when data are considered for secondary use. These include the fact that priorities at the time of registration will be aligned with the clinician's or administrative needs, as well as other factors related to the patient's behaviour during visits, including loss of follow-up, missing information, data inconsistencies, and others [99].

1.5.2 Electronic Health Records: Advantages and Challenges

The reuse of EHRs has emerged as a transformative practice with multifaceted advantages, influencing the clinical, organizational, and societal dimensions of healthcare. At the clinical level, the repurposing of EHRs has substantially improved the quality of care and contributed to the reduction of medical errors, showcasing tangible benefits for patients. From an organizational standpoint, EHR reuse has positively impacted financial and operational performance, underscoring its potential to streamline healthcare processes. Specifically, the use of EHR data was also found to expedite healthcare quality measurements. Unlike standard quality measures, electronic aggregation of patient data can accelerate analysis and lead to better results among standard quality measures. More than 250 studies that were included in a qualitative synthesis reported that the utilization of EHRs led to improved protocol adherence, large-scale clinical monitoring, and decreased adverse medication events [101]. Together with standardized quality measures, EHRs can also facilitate the formulation of new quality measures such as those that are more continuous (e.g. actual blood pressure measures) and not only binary (e.g. when blood pressure checking is performed or when it is below/above a specific threshold) [102]. Moreover, the secondary use of EHRs has facilitated superior research, promising advancements in population health [99]. EHR data reuse can facilitate the design of retrospective studies by using existing data pools. It will also accelerate patient enrolment in prospective studies, thereby substantially reducing the costs associated with patient recruitment [103]. Since EHRs include a wide array of data (such as laboratory data, vital signs, and other clinical parameters), they can also enable patient monitoring by examining a wide array of health outcomes [104]. Compared with traditional means of data collection, the use of EHR data also offers public health benefits such as individual telephone- or paper-based reporting. This enables public health officials to perform rapid monitoring of the spread and emergence of diseases [102]. Finally, EHR data can support decision-making processes related to medical products by facilitating safety monitoring. For example, in the United States, the FDA relies on aggregated EHR data to perform safety evaluations of FDA-regulated products—namely drugs and medical devices [102].

However, navigating the landscape of EHR reuse is not without its challenges. The issue of representativeness poses a significant concern, particularly when the geographical areas providing data fail to accurately represent the targeted population for inference. Furthermore, inaccuracies or limitations in data pertaining to socioeconomic status, race, ethnicity, and other crucial factors may impede the reliability of the findings. The original design of EHRs for clinical and administrative purposes introduces challenges related to data availability and interpretation. Insufficient recording of factors relevant for addressing social and behavioural determinants of health (SBDH) and reducing inequalities diminishes the data's potential for research purposes, as it may be hindered by various forms of bias. Additionally, the presence of unstructured data, such as adverse events and symptoms, necessitates advancements in technologies such as natural language processing for more effective analysis [105].

A critical gap exists in current EHRs concerning key research factors, which are designed primarily for billing and scheduling rather than for epidemiological research. Variables crucial for understanding socioeconomic status and SBDH factors are often absent, limiting the comprehensive use of EHR data for research purposes. Visit censoring, where visits are not seamlessly connected between different health facilities, introduces challenges such as right or left censorship, impacting the continuity of patient records, for example, when patients are referred to a new centre without previous clinical information [100].

Security and privacy concerns surround the reuse of EHRs. The vulnerability of EHRs to cyber threats has raised alarms, necessitating ongoing efforts to implement cryptographic, noncryptographic, and hybrid access control models and blockchain technology for data protection. Furthermore, cases of ambiguity in the question of data ownership may cause privacy issues, with patients consenting not only for the use of their data but also for the existence of a wide spectrum of data uses that may be included in this consent without the patient truly acknowledging it. In fact, obtaining explicit consent for every secondary use has been catalogued as time-consuming, costly, and exhausting. Additionally, the existence of previous events, which have led to data leaks, illicit or illegal data selling or loss, makes the trust relationship between patients and data primary users or collectors difficult [99].

Moreover, the discrepancies between the General Data Protection Regulation (GDPR) principles and the objectives of EHRs pose a regulatory challenge in the EU, as the principles may limit data collection and use, conflicting with the broader goals of secondary health data utilization. The GDPR defines six main data protection principles: (1) lawfulness, fairness, and transparency; (2) purpose limitations; (3) data minimization; (4) accuracy; (5) storage limitations; and (6) integrity and confidentiality. In the case of EHR, these principles can contradict the characteristics and objectives of EHR, as if followed to the rule, these principles generally mean that healthcare data collection should be limited, together with its use, and deleted immediately after its purpose has been achieved. In the case of secondary health data, almost all antagonist principles are promoted, as more data would mean more potential for epidemiological research and other purposes, which would increase its potential. Its secondary use is also encouraged for institutions and individuals to serve as tools for healthcare improvement, and ultimately, secondary use is necessary for this purpose [99].

Dilatory regulations, such as the Health Insurance Portability and Accountability Act (HIPAA) and Health Information Technology for Economic and Clinical Health (HITECH) Act applied in the United States, face a widening gap with rapidly advancing technologies. Patient expectations for immediate data availability clash with regulations that do not meet present-day requirements. Emerging scenarios, such as the integration of social media platforms into health data, challenge outdated regulations, emphasizing the need for flexible and adaptive regulatory frameworks to keep pace with evolving health data and EHR usage [99]. In essence, while the advantages of EHR reuse are substantial, addressing these challenges is crucial for unlocking its full potential in the dynamic landscape of secondary health data utilization.

The recent EHDS regulation [106] establishes that in the European Union, certain categories of health data, such as EHRs, are registered in electronic format systematically and according to specific data quality requirements (defined by means of implementing acts adopted by the European Commission) to contribute to the high quality and continuity of healthcare. The European electronic health record exchange format forms the basis for specifications related to the registration and exchange of electronic health data, which will be accessible for secondary use across the Union through a common mechanism for the purpose of creating scientific, innovative, and societal value.

1.5.3   Electronic Health Records: Examples of Reuse

1.5.3.1   The Use of EHR Data in Research

EHRs have become invaluable in various realms of healthcare, highlighting their versatility in the secondary use of health data. In the domain of clinical research, EHRs play a pivotal role in designing and conducting clinical trials for new medicines, addressing the shortage of trained medical staff in healthcare organizations and facilitating the exploration of new or enhanced drugs to meet evolving healthcare needs [107]. Leveraging existing patient data, EHRs contribute to predicting diseases, investigating drug behaviours across different diseases or patient profiles, and even aiding in the development of vaccines [108–110]. EHR data can also be utilized to identify new uses for existing medicine, with the aim of enabling a rapid and cost-effective approach to drug (re)discovery. For example, a genetically informed drug-repurposing pipeline that can be used in diabetes management has been developed and investigated. Among the 20 candidate drug–gene pairs validated, angiotensin-converting enzyme inhibitors and calcium channel blockers (CCBs) showed evidence of glycaemic regulation involvement. CCBs were found to be strong candidates for both reducing blood glucose levels and managing cardiovascular disease [111]. Furthermore, retrospective analyses of EHR data can reveal potential contributing factors that might cause certain adverse health outcomes such as prolonged postoperative opioid use in opioid-naïve patients. Several independent predictors of prolonged postoperative opioid use, such as alcohol abuse, black race, Medicaid insurance, diabetes, mood disorders, hypertension, and chronic kidney disease, can be investigated via perioperative patient screening, providing education to patients and clinicians, and performing close postoperative follow-up, among other methods [112].

1.5.3.2   The Use of EHR Data in Public Health

The utility of EHR data extends to public health surveillance (PHS), where it automates surveillance processes to identify potential outbreaks efficiently and prevent their escalation [113]. This application has proven effective not only in developed countries such as the UK, the United States, France, Norway, Canada, and Australia [114] but also in developing nations when necessary [115]. Public health agencies, including the US Centers for Disease Control and Prevention (CDC), have started utilizing EHR data. In 2003, the CDC launched the BioSense system to quickly identify bioterrorism-related illnesses [116]. Since then, BioSense's network has grown to include 1700 hospitals, and its mission has expanded beyond bioterrorism. Currently, BioSense is the only nationwide surveillance system in the United States that integrates local, regional, and national data to monitor all health-related threats. Consequently, through initiatives such as BioSense, the CDC can use EHR data to track and address various public health issues, from the emergence of influenza H1N1 to an anthrax attack [116]. The global impact of the COVID-19 outbreak further underscored the importance of digital data recording systems, such as EHRs, in enhancing public health responses and preparedness [117].

1.5.3.3   The Use of EHR Data in Quality Management

In the realms of clinical audit and quality assurance, EHRs provide a wealth of accurate and detailed information that is essential for systematically setting standards, analysing data, and monitoring performance to maintain high-quality standards. The use of EHR data in clinical audits not only streamlines the auditing process for greater convenience but also contributes to improving the quality of care delivered to patients [118]. For example, by implementing computer-based standing orders, the Regenstrief Institute in Indianapolis increased the pneumococcal vaccination rate, a standard quality measure, from 31% to 51% [119]. Timely and effective quality measurement via EHR data will allow institutions to identify and address shortcomings in real time rather than respond retrospectively. For example, the rate of deep venous thrombosis/pulmonary embolism (from 8.2% to 4.9%) in Partners' healthcare in Boston nearly halved when computerized alerts were used for anticoagulation prophylaxis [120]. Another example is the Geisinger Health System in Danville, Pennsylvania, which uses its EHR system to monitor performance continuously on the basis of various standard and internal quality metrics. This approach has elevated nearly all its quality indicators above national averages and enhanced the quality of care across 32 performance measures evaluated in Medicare's Physician Group Practice Demonstration Initiative. These measures include diabetes, congestive heart failure, coronary artery disease, and preventive care [121–123].

The examples of EHR reuse presented in clinical research, public health surveillance, and clinical audit and quality assurance collectively highlight the transformative impact of EHRs in enhancing healthcare delivery, research, and response capabilities.

1.6 Human Genomic, Proteomic Data

1.6.1 Genomic and Proteomic Data: Background

Two decades ago, the invention of spotting oligonucleotide probes at a high density to glass or nylon arrays transformed the study of gene expression and accelerated the adoption of bioinformatics as an important element of biological studies [124]. The term "proteomics" was coined in the mid-1990s to describe the comprehensive study of a proteome, which encompasses the proteins expressed by a genome. This field involves large-scale analysis of proteins, namely examination of protein expression, structure, modifications, functions, and interactions [125]. Proteomics is a crucial postgenomic approach for enhancing the understanding of gene function [126]. On the other hand, human genomic data, according to the FDA, are data that can be obtained from germline sources (inherited from parents), somatic sources (e.g. mutations in tumour tissues), or mitochondrial sources (e.g. for tracing maternal lineages). Biological samples from humans may also contain nonhuman genomic molecules, such as microbial DNA or other potentially infectious agents. The type of genomic data produced depends on the analytes and the technology platforms used [127].

Currently, new research into how genetic variants affect health and disease has been conducted through the mapping of the human genome. Diseases such as diabetes, Alzheimer's disease, cardiovascular disease, and others are not being studied in relation to genetic variants for what has become part of a "personalized medicine" approach aimed at improving patient care. Institutions have been developed for this purpose. Community efforts include the Microarray Gene Expression Data (MGED) Society in 1999 and the Gene Ontology (GO) standard vocabulary. Other more recent efforts include the eMERGE network (2007), which is a consortium that integrates this innovation pathway, explores the utility of DNA repositories and electronic medical records (EMRs) to promote advancements in genomic science, and offers an initial step in the creation of data-driven strategies to integrate genomic data into standard healthcare delivery [128]. Gene Expression Omnibus (GEO) and

ArrayExpress are also part of this attempt to increase innovation in the field. Another EU initiative is very important: "1+ Million Genomes" (1+MG) seeks to provide secure access to genomic data and associated clinical information across Europe. It aims to advance cutting-edge research, inform health policy decisions, and promote personalized healthcare treatments that have the potential to enhance disease prevention. As one of the largest global genomic projects, 1+MG plays a crucial role in establishing international standards in the field of genomics [129].

1.6.2   Genomic and Proteomic Data: Advantages and Challenges

The utilization of publicly available genomic and proteomic data holds substantial advantages for both the scientific community and individual researchers [130]. Sharing research data with the public and storing them in dedicated databases with backup mechanisms can prevent information loss, addressing the heightened risk associated with storing data on private computers and servers. Notable repositories, such as the Sequence Read Archive (SRA)/European Nucleotide Archive (ENA) and Gene Expression Omnibus (GEO), offer secure platforms for genomic and gene expression data. Beyond safeguarding against loss, the reuse of such data fosters scientific progress and discovery [131]. For example, integrating diverse data sources, such as exRNA metadata and biomedical ontologies, via linked data technologies can enhance the generation and interpretation of hypotheses within independent biological contexts [132]. The transformative potential of reusing data in medicine extends to reshaping medical service practices, making the benefits of data reuse outweigh the associated risks [133, 134]. Additionally, the reuse of genomic and proteomic data has proven to be a strategic approach for addressing gaps in biomedical research and establishing starting points for experimental medical investigations [133]. Furthermore, this approach maximizes efficiency in terms of time, labour, and cost, offering economical alternatives to overcoming methodological constraints in conducting new experiments [135]. Critically, the sharing of datasets not only benefits the scientific community and society but also provides advantages for authors themselves [136–138]. Researchers can build reputations by publishing high-quality datasets while sharing these datasets enhances research visibility and increases the likelihood of additional citations. The surge in data reuse also underscores the growing need for larger databases, exemplified by the exponential growth of repositories such as the SRA and GenBank, which have expanded rapidly in size over just a few years [139–141].

Reusing biological data presents formidable challenges, as outlined by several documented hurdles. First, a substantial investment in infrastructure and software development remains imperative for effective data reuse. Scientists currently grapple with the need to navigate diverse proteomics resources to gather comprehensive information about a given protein. Despite facilitating the connection process between omics datasets through sample identifiers, traditional repositories are often field specific such as genomics or proteomics. This proves to be limiting in the face of growing interdisciplinary research that integrates various omics sciences [142]. Major institutions such as the European Bioinformatics Institute (EBI) and National Center for Biotechnology Information (NCBI) have established specific databases for BioSamples [143] to facilitate the linking of different studies conducted using the same sample. Additionally, proteomics data are complex per se because of alternative splicing, PTMs, and protein degradation events, as well as the interconnectivity of proteins into complexes and signalling networks that are prone to changes in time and space [144]. Addressing this complexity requires new analytical and bioinformatics methodologies on an annual basis [145, 146], introducing further complications to data standardization and deposition. Furthermore, since the proteomics audience includes a variety of different roles (e.g. biologists who investigate protein mechanisms or computational biologists who develop new software for facilitating analysis and data interpretation) [147], data sharing in proteomics thus necessitates substantial investment and infrastructure. Because of this, there is a growing consensus on the need for public dissemination of proteomics data. In addition, in comparison with genomics, proteomic public data remain less common, thus still requiring substantial investment and infrastructure. Current projects in the proteomics field include the recent ProteomeXchange (PX) consortium, the Global Proteome Machine Database (GPBDB) [148], PeptideAtlas [149], and the Proteomics Identification Database (PRIDE) [150]. Other initiatives, such as Peptidome [151] and Tranche [152], are now discontinued due to a lack of funding, which negatively impacts data sharing in this field. The sheer multitude of data types and formats adds another layer of complexity to the task at hand. Ideally, repositories should not only house data but also ensure that it is linked to quality control (QC) metrics. Moreover, the generation of these metrics should ideally occur simultaneously with data acquisition in the laboratory. A critical challenge lies in the absence of experimental and technical metadata, particularly concerning proteomics, hindering effective data reuse in scientific endeavours. Finally, the identification of false positives in large datasets and when combining different datasets remains a problem [149, 153]. Therefore, protein expression resources should conduct the most thorough statistical analyses possible.

1.6.3 Genomic and Proteomic Data: Examples of Reuse

The Use of Genomic and Proteomic Data for Research

One avenue involves the reuse of raw genomic and proteomic data for novel biological investigations. For example, a dataset comprising 81 samples from white blood cells and 1463 from various organs, measured on the Affymetrix HG U133A platform, facilitated a study examining the correspondence in their expression profiles [154]. The results revealed significant overlap in the transcriptomes of white blood cells and other organs, which aligns with the understanding that most genes are expressed across various tissues [155]. Expression data were also employed to pinpoint the tissue of origin for metastatic cancers lacking a known primary site, leveraging classifiers trained on a vast dataset encompassing 5577 samples from 56 cancer types and 1667 normal samples from 44 tissues [156]. These examples underscore how large and diverse datasets can provide profound insights, particularly in studies where global transcriptomic profiles enable comparisons across different cellular states.

The Use of Genomic and Proteomic Data for Conducting Meta-Analyses
Data reuse also involves the utilization of public data for conducting meta-analyses of summary data. Meta-analyses, which use summary-level data, offer a popular and flexible approach to repurposing existing data from various array platforms. Gene expression data have been subjected to meta-analysis for an array of biological inquiries, with emerging studies employing this technique on public datasets to discern signals that are not readily apparent in individual datasets [157–159]. Noteworthy examples include a study analysing 324 differentially expressed genes in individuals with Down syndrome, drawn from case–control data across 45 studies [160]. In the context of cancer research, microarray data from ArrayExpress, GEO, and Oncomine datasets were amalgamated to identify urinary biomarkers specific to prostate cancer [161].

The Integration with Other Omics Datasets
The integration of proteomics datasets with other public omics datasets opens new avenues for data scientists. Proteogenomics, a methodology employed in cancer studies, focuses on cancer-specific peptides with diagnostic and therapeutic potential. The Clinical Proteomic Tumor Analysis Consortium (CPTAC) of the US National Cancer Institute (NCI) has published impactful studies on various tumours, including colorectal, breast, and ovarian cancers [162–164]. This integration of proteomics with other omics datasets underscores the potential for cross-disciplinary insights and advancements in understanding complex biological phenomena.

1.7 National Registries

1.7.1 National Registries: Background

The term "patient registry" typically refers to registries focused on health information, distinguishing them from other types of record sets, although there is no universally accepted definition. E.M. Brooke, in a 1974 World Health Organization publication, described registries in health information systems as "a file of documents containing uniform information about individual persons, collected in a systematic and comprehensive way, in order to serve a predetermined purpose" [165]. The US National Committee on Vital and Health Statistics describes registries used for various purposes in public health and medicine as "an organized system for collecting, storing, retrieving, analysing, and disseminating information on individuals who either have a particular disease, a condition (e.g., a risk factor) that predisposes them to a health-related event, or prior exposure to substances (or circumstances) known or suspected to cause adverse health effects" [166].

In the case of national registries, these are created with the objective of collecting data to measure progress, drive action, prevent disease, improve health, and ultimately improve health for all people [167]. Registries tend to be composed of data from multiple sources that are linked by a specific methodology, i.e. direct chart abstraction by trained data abstractors, who tend to work within a coordination centre at the registry. This data collection tends to be guided by a manual that defines the data elements, which are usually categorized as demographics, operative data, hospitalizations, follow-up, etc. [168].

Multiple national registries exist worldwide, focusing on different diseases, patient groups, and demographic characteristics of patients. Key infrastructure is necessary for national registries to promote interoperability; as an example, the rare disease network for care and research in France, established as a part of the first national plan for rare diseases (2005–2008), is based on a three-pillar architecture composed of (1) the definition of a national patient ID, (2) the definition of a common data format compatible with EHR standards, and (3) security [169].

1.7.2 National Registries Worldwide: Advantages and Challenges

National registries can collect large amounts of data (e.g. the registry provided by the Michigan Arthroplasty Registry Collaborative Quality Initiative [MARCQI] contains more than 375,000 cases), which can be collected from multiple sources and supplemented with other types of data (e.g. administrative billing data) [168]. National registries enable state-level collaboration. While in other cases, surgeons and hospitals compete in between, here, they engage in open data sharing and cooperate on quality improvement projects. The value of registries can be exemplified by the fact that they usually collect data from multiple institutions, making EHR and clinical databases the only components of a population registry [170]. In contrast to clinical databases, which do not require strict definitions of common features, this is mandatory for registries [170]. Furthermore, registries aim to collect the highest number of cases (if possible, in total), which makes them a representative data source for a defined population [165, 170, 171]. Registries also perform a constant update of the patient status by following a predefined schedule [170]. In addition, medical registries collect data in a way that allows comparisons of the results at the national (or even higher) level. Given that national medical registries are usually focused on a disease of interest, they fit their predefined purpose and collect specified outcomes [171], which makes them more uniform than EHR registries, for example. Taking the domain of cancer as an example, the primary goal of the cancer national registry is to record all new cancer cases that arise within a defined population by focusing on epidemiology and public health practices [172]. These registries are rich sources of information on the cancer burden that can be used for healthcare planning and evaluation purposes and for conducting studies on prevention, early detection/screening, and cancer-related healthcare, which are used by epidemiologists and public health planners [16]. These concepts can be applied equally to other disease paradigms.

Registry data pose several challenges, encompassing issues related to data completeness, accuracy, and scope. First, ensuring data completeness is a persistent challenge, as demonstrated by the MARCQI, where reported cases are compared with validated statewide administrative billing data to confirm completeness. The extensive time and labour required for data abstraction on a large scale can result in substantial lag times between case performance and result reporting, prompting some registries to set specific time limits for data abstraction. Additionally, the scope and definition of data elements at the registry level may impose limitations. Another limitation arises from the fact that data are captured only for patients treated within institutions affiliated with the specific registry. Furthermore, the accuracy of registry data is compromised by potential inaccuracies in the coding process, as well as errors caused by programming and inaccurate transcription [173]. One of the pitfalls of registry data is nonstandardized and inactive follow-up, which may lead to incomplete and inaccurate outcomes. In certain cases, the follow-up is performed in a passive manner by using linkages with administrative databases. However, since the primary aim of these datasets is not for research purposes, these methods may introduce errors due to misclassification of outcomes resulting from coding errors and different coding practices. Additionally, the passive nature of data collection can lead to missing data, which can hinder further analysis in research practice. Finally, one should bear in mind that data entry into a registry is not strictly monitored, which may create the possibility that ineligible patients enter the registry and thus introduce bias in the findings obtained from registry data analysis. Therefore, registry data, like all other RWD, require careful monitoring, quality assessments, and validations so that they provide reliable results that can be applied to the population of interest [174]. Collectively, these challenges contribute to analytical limitations and hinder the ability to establish causality via registry data [168].

1.7.3   National Registries Worldwide: Examples of Reuse

1.7.3.1   The Use of National Registry Data in Public Health Research at the National and International Levels

The secondary use of health data, particularly those harnessed from national registries, represents a transformative force in addressing diverse health-related questions and guiding public health initiatives. National registries worldwide have become powerful reservoirs of health data, offering a wealth of information for diverse research endeavours. In 2020, data from a National Cancer Centre in Japan were harnessed to explore the correlation between airborne pollen levels and cancer incidence. A significant association between elevated pollen levels measured two years prior and the incidence of breast cancer and other forms of cancer was revealed, highlighting the potential of national registries in uncovering environmental factors impacting health [175].

Further examples underscore the versatility of national registry data. The Lithuanian Compulsory Health Insurance Information System database, SVEIDRA, was used to support the hypothesis that patients with rheumatic diseases face a higher risk of mortality and lower life expectancy than the general population does. A total of 11,636 patients and a follow-up period of 43,064.34 person-years were included, and 950 registered deaths were identified, emphasizing the utility of national registry data for exploring disease-specific mortality risks [176]. Additionally, the National Arthroplasty Registry served as a valuable resource for a comparative observational study involving 581,818 procedures. Compared with procedures employing technology-assisted instrumentation, there was a noteworthy association between conventional instrumentation during total knee arthroplasty and early postoperative death, highlighting the potential of registry data to inform best practices in healthcare procedures [177]. A comprehensive population-based nationwide cohort study conducted in Finland, which utilized data from two national health registries, examined 933,823 children born between 1996 and 2011. This study investigated potential infections with *C. trachomatis*, revealing a rare occurrence rate of 0.22 per 1000 births. These findings challenge previous assumptions, shedding light on transmission dynamics during pregnancy and illustrating the ability of national registries to provide statistically significant answers to common clinical questions [178]. The impact of different dialysis modalities was addressed by drawing on data from national and regional registries of ten countries (Australia, New Zealand, Japan, China, Taiwan, Korea, Thailand, Hong Kong, Malaysia, and India). Despite challenges such as varying coding techniques and data limitations, data from 201,590 patients were useful for identifying significant influencing factors between dialysis modalities and outcomes [179].

1.7.3.2 The Use of National Registry Data for Worldwide Collaboration

The National Cardiovascular Data Registry (NCDR), established by the American College of Cardiology, stands as an exemplary source of standardized, evidence-based data on clinical topics and cardiovascular procedures [180, 181]. Another illustrative example arises from the multinational network of diabetic care centres known as SWEET. A 2021 study within this network utilized linear and logistic regression models to analyse participant data, revealing that lower HbA1c levels and fewer diabetic ketoacidosis (DKA) episodes were observed in participants utilizing insulin pumps, continuous glucose monitoring, or a combination of both [182]. The collaborative nature of registries, exemplified by initiatives such as the SWEET, fosters international collaboration, enabling the evaluation of information from small national populations on a global scale, the establishment of benchmarking practices, and the synergistic effects of shared data [183]. Other examples of this collaboration of data between registries include the collaboration between ten national registries to evaluate the outcome of renal replacement therapy for diabetic neuropathy, suggesting the flexibility of research options that could be derived from international data use [184]. Finally, a collaborative project involving 7 well-known registries and the SWEET initiative provided a comparative perspective, combining data from over 900 facilities and 100,000 paediatric patients. This collaboration not only grants access to updated and representative data but also fosters open benchmarking collaboration between registries [183]. Collaborative initiatives among registries worldwide further amplify the potential of data management, allowing for the analysis of large datasets that were previously impractical for researchers.

1.7.3.3   The Use of National Registries for Supporting Regulatory Assessments

When RCT data are unavailable or are not ethical or feasible (as in the case of many rare diseases), patient registry data may support regulatory decision-making. For haemophilia, for example, the updated guideline for factor VIII products published by the EMA removes the obligation to conduct clinical trials in treatment-naïve patients but requires postlicensing trials on the basis of key data elements collected in patient registries [185]. Additionally, as in other European Medicines Agency (EMA) reviews, for conditional marketing authorization products, registration studies can provide postlicensing data that meet specific regulatory obligations to confirm safety and/or efficacy, such as for the recently approved chimeric antigen receptor (CAR) T-cell product thiagenlecleucel and axicabtagene in siloleucel [186, 187]. Certain registries may be particularly valuable in terms of the size and representativeness of the patient population, the length of follow-up of medically exposed patients, and the availability of data not collected by other real-world repositories.

The wealth of insights derived from these examples collectively underscores the pivotal role of national registries in advancing our understanding of health dynamics and in shaping evidence-based interventions, highlighting the substantial impact and diverse applications of national registries in advancing our understanding of health-related phenomena at both the national scale and the international scale.

1.8   Person-Generated Electronic Health Data

1.8.1   *Person-Generated Health Data: Background*

Information on health generated by patients is not a new concept. Instead, oral medical history has always served as the basis of medical consultation. Recently, this data collection process has also required the storage of records of medical events, i.e. symptom frequency, blood glucose concentration records, to provide a longitudinal record that will assist in clinical diagnosis and management.

The Office of the National Coordinator for Health Information Technology (ONC) from the United States defined person-generated health data (PGHD) as "health-related data including health history, symptoms, biometric data, treatment history, lifestyle choices, and other information-created, recorded, gathered or inferred by or from patients or their designees" [188]. PGHD differs from data produced in clinical settings and provider encounters in two important ways. First, patients, not providers, are primarily responsible for collecting or maintaining this information. Second, patients direct the sharing of this information with healthcare providers and other stakeholders. In this way, PGHD complements the provider's collection and flow of health information in the health system. PGHD includes various data types, such as the following:

- Vital signs measured by the patient (or proxy) (e.g. temperature, blood pressure, blood glucose, weight), which can be captured manually, by reading a mechanical or electronic device, or automatically via a monitoring device.
- Self-reported lifestyle data (e.g. caloric intake, diet, exercise, hydration, and medication adherence) that are recorded by the patient or family member, and data collection usually occurs manually.
- Self-reported as perceived quality of life data (e.g. mood, sleep quality, level of pain, social contacts), which are mainly captured manually by the patient or a patient proxy.
- Other data, apart from health-related data, are known to the provider by the patient on a personalized individual basis [188].

PGHD collection can be supported by different tools, including smartphone apps, wearables, sensors, smart home appliances, medical record apps, etc. [189]. Although diverse organizations, such as the Veterans Health Administration, Kaiser Permanente, and others, are promoting a more systematic use of PGHD in its early stage, further work is still needed on many aspects of the PHGD to achieve its full potential.

1.8.2 Person-Generated Health Data: Advantages and Challenges

Person-generated health data (PGHD) have emerged as a dynamic source with notable advantages and challenges in the realm of secondary health data use. One key advantage lies in its capacity to be recorded outside of clinical settings, significantly extending potential data collection timeframes [190]. PGHD is valuable because it can be recorded outside of a clinical or laboratory setting in places where people spend most of their time (e.g. at home, in the office, or in their community). PGHD may also be measured more frequently than conventional medical data. PGHD can be combined with medical and other data (such as geographic location, weather, and community events) to provide a more detailed picture of an individual's health over time [190].

By using digital tools to collect PGHD, researchers can communicate more widely and directly with potential study participants, allowing them to collect more data and improve their workflow. Special techniques include the use of scientific data platforms and remote sensing. Researchers can expand recruitment and enrolment in their studies by incorporating digital tools that incorporate PGHD into their study designs and protocols, such as mobile health devices, online discussion forums, and health information platforms. Researchers do not need to rely as much on relationships with physicians or health systems to identify potential study participants. Instead, they could provide promotional information about their studies directly to a broader and perhaps more diverse patient population through online postings on social media and email lists [191]. The use of PGHD technologies for electronic data collection and transmission helps streamline the research flow. Instead of manually entering patient data, data can flow electronically into the research database. Tools capable of cleaning data can simplify the process of ensuring that the data are complete and ready for analysis. These electronic processes reduce the amount of work required by researchers and reduce the potential for human error in data entry [192].

PGHD has also proven invaluable in the context of clinical trials, especially in the reporting of adverse events. Patient reported Outcomes (PROs) derived from PGHD offer a more accurate portrayal of adverse events, addressing the significant underreporting—up to 76%—observed in traditional clinical trials. This clarity in reporting, whether through the support of data or digital twins during clinical trials or the utilization of other sources of information post-product release based on PGHD, enhances the understanding of patient experiences and contributes to the overall assessment of interventions [193].

The large volume of health data generated on a continuous basis provides a plethora of opportunities for secondary uses and for gathering new scientific evidence that can impact the population.

The integration of PGHD into healthcare practices also introduces a set of challenges that necessitate careful consideration in the secondary use of health data. One primary challenge is associated with data governance, given that PGHD involves data generated directly by patients. Clear definitions regarding data holders and providers, the process of data collection, and establishing agreements between stakeholders become imperative for effective and ethical information collection [189]. The incorporation of new sources of data collection, such as the utilization of social media for pharmaco-epidemiologic research, presents an additional ethical consideration that requires thoughtful examination [189]. Motivating patients to actively engage as data providers poses another challenge, with concerns arising regarding unclear motivations and potential reluctance [189]. Additionally, patients can be inconsistent with using their apps and wearables, which introduces a new source of bias to the data [194].

Moreover, the storage and management of PGHD currently demand substantial resources, posing a risk of deteriorating the doctor–patient relationship and rendering the data difficult to interpret [104]. The delineation of clear responsibilities and liabilities is crucial to address potential issues arising from the use of inaccurate PGHD in diagnosis or treatment. This includes establishing accountability for errors, whether they originate from the patient, the app used for data collection, or other contributing factors [195]. Apps and wearables may use different tools and methods for data collection, thereby affecting the reliability and accuracy of the data [190]. Further complications to data accuracy and reliability are introduced by the participants' lack of knowledge. For example, they may incorrectly capture self-reported data (such as that related to anxiety) if they do not receive proper education upfront [196]. In addition to patients, practitioners may also misinterpret PGHD, and in some cases, PGHD lacks context (e.g. a spike in heart rate may be caused by exercise or stress); in both cases, the interpretation of the results may be misleading [197]. Additionally, the diverse characteristics of PGHD, encompassing various items, tools, communication channels, and workflows, necessitate the development of new standards to meet the demands of multiple stakeholders, including patients, app developers, EHR suppliers, and physicians [195]. Finally, data governance is an essential part of the effective use of PGHD and is required at every stage of the process, from data collection to dissemination of results. Agreement between study organizers and participants on the principles of information sharing is central to ensuring trust and includes consideration of confidentiality and legal liability. The development of patient privacy standards and guidelines and/or the updating of existing guidelines [198, 199] is important as the use of PGHD increases and new issues emerge. Legal aspects such as informed consent and data security are a concern in PGHD research, as are standards for electronic consent (consent is evolving) [200]. As the healthcare landscape evolves with the integration of PGHD, addressing these challenges becomes imperative to ensure the responsible and effective use of PGHD for improving healthcare outcomes.

1.8.3 PGHD: Examples of Reuse

The Use of PGHD in Research Endeavours
The secondary use of person-generated health data (PGHD) occurs in various domains, demonstrating its versatility and impact on biomedical research and healthcare practices. In the realm of scientific initiatives, the US Precision Medicine Initiative (PMI), specifically the All of Us Research Program [201], underscores the importance of collecting primary PGHD through participatory technologies such as web-based surveys, wearable devices, and smartphone apps. This ambitious programme aims to build a vast data repository with over one million participants, collaborating with projects such as the health US-based eHeart Study [202] and the Health Data Exploration Network [203] to collect primary PGHD reporting

environmental risk factors for biomedical research across diverse populations of both healthy individuals and patients.

Biometric data, encompassing wireless scales, blood pressure cuffs, thermometers, pulse oximeters, heart rate monitors, and blood glucose metres offer valuable insights when integrated with smartphone apps [204–206]. Some smartwatches even include electrocardiogram readings, which are more accurate than ambulatory ECGs and are useful for screening for atrial fibrillation and cardiac issues. The reuse of biometric data highlights the potential of PGHD in monitoring and managing various health parameters. Physical activity monitoring has evolved from accelerometers in the 1980s [207] to modern wrist-worn activity trackers, which have gained acceptance in research due to enhanced data accuracy [208–210]. Smartphones equipped with accelerometers can distinguish between different physical activities, offering a convenient and acceptable alternative to wrist-based trackers [211, 212]. Given the established benefits of regular physical activity, the use of PGHD from these devices holds promise for future studies.

The Use of Substandard Real-Time PGHD Data for Detecting and Predicting Health-Related Outcomes
Location data, derived from smartphones via GPS, Wi-Fi, and Google Location History, provide insights into patients' community mobility and its correlation with mental and physical well-being [213–216]. Such data can offer valuable information about daily activities outside the home, contributing to the assessment of quality of life. In mental health studies, GPS measurements of movement have been employed to detect depression with a remarkable accuracy of 87% [217].

The Use of PGHD in Decision-Making Processes
The use of technological innovations for PGHD has the potential to improve the individualized management of disease care (such as cancer) across the continuum from primary prevention to treatment and survival [218]. For example, a PGHD analysis focused on the detection of mental distress facilitated the identification of individuals in need of mental health treatment, help, and support [219]. Mobile technology applications that allow patients to identify and report symptoms or side effects of treatment between routine clinic visits can improve adherence to treatment plans [220].

The Use of PGHD to Improve the Collection of Certain Data Types
The assessment of dietary habits, a historically challenging endeavour, has improved with PGHD. Traditional retrospective questionnaires suffer from recall and social desirability biases. Web- or app-based dietary measurements provide a more accurate and less burdensome alternative [221, 222]. Future innovations may involve the use of smartphone cameras and machine learning algorithms to identify foods and portions, reducing participant burden and enhancing the collection of dietary information in studies [223, 224]. These examples illustrate the expansive potential of PGHD in transforming healthcare research and practices across diverse domains.

1.9   Social and Behavioural Determinants of Health

1.9.1   Social and Behavioural Determinants of Health: Background

The Healthy People programme, which is part of the US Department of Health and Human Services Office of Disease Prevention and Health Promotion, defines social determinants of health (SDOHs) as "the conditions in the environments where people are born, live, learn, work, play, worship, and age that affect a wide range of health, functioning, and quality-of-life outcomes and risks" [225]. SDOHs are also known as social and behavioural determinants of health (SBDHs) [226]. As stated by the WHO, the SDOH has important implications for health inequalities, namely unfair and avoidable differences in health status within and between countries. In countries of all income levels, health and disease follow a social gradient: the worse the socioeconomic status is, the worse the health. It is estimated that social factors may be more important than healthcare or lifestyle choices in influencing health. For example, many studies have shown that SDOH is responsible for 30–55% of health effects. Another estimation shows that sectors outside health contribute to population health outcomes to a greater extent than does the health sector itself [227].

With respect to five key areas: (1) economic stability, (2) education access and quality, (3) social and community context, (4) neighbourhood and environment, and (5) healthcare access and quality, research has demonstrated that SBDH factors account for more than one-third of the estimated annual deaths in the United States. In contrast, integrating SBDH factors such as education, lifestyle, physical activity, and diet could improve the management of diseases such as Alzheimer's disease or diabetes. Integrating SBDH into the EHR system could help address such a factor's key role in healthcare and further improve patient care outcomes in ways that would not be possible otherwise [226].

1.9.2   SBDH: Advantages and Challenges

The secondary use of social determinants of health (SBDH) data presents notable advantages and challenges, as recognized in the literature. Reusing SBDH data has the potential to significantly enhance care management by incorporating economic, social, and behavioural factors associated with a patient's health. This holistic approach to decision-making improves the efficiency of care plans and better addresses the needs of vulnerable populations, ensuring a more comprehensive and tailored healthcare strategy [228]. Moreover, addressing SBDH factors has the potential to reduce healthcare utilization, as exemplified by programmes initiated by the Centres for Medicare and Medicaid. These initiatives aim to systematically identify and address health-related social needs, such as food insecurity and inadequate housing, with the goal of lowering the overall demand for healthcare services

among community-dwelling Medicare and Medicaid beneficiaries [229]. Such programmes signify a transformative shift in how clinical and community service providers collaborate, ensuring that patients receive services and support aligned with
their specific needs.

Furthermore, the integration of SBDH data holds promise for improving risk
adjustment payment models and enhancing the design of performance-based incentives. Notably, the first US payment model incorporating SBDH variables,
MassHealth, introduced variables such as a neighbourhood stress score and a measure of unstable housing. The inclusion of these variables, alongside additional data
such as individuals' use of services from the Departments of Mental Health or
Developmental Services, in the diagnosis-based model resulted in a more accurate
alignment of payments to costs for several vulnerable categories. This example
highlights the potential of SBDH data to refine payment models and incentivize
performance in a manner that considers the diverse social determinants impacting
healthcare outcomes [230]. In essence, the reuse of SBDH data offers a multifaceted
approach to healthcare management, with the potential to optimize care plans,
reduce healthcare utilization, and enhance the alignment of payments to actual
costs, particularly for vulnerable populations.

Reusing SBDH data presents several challenges that warrant attention and
thoughtful solutions. First and foremost, data collection and algorithm bias pose
significant risks. Currently, the representation of SBDH in EHRs is limited, with
only some aspects registered in clinical text. The integration of SBDH data with
technologies such as AI to support clinical decisions holds promise but is suscepti-
ble to bias, potentially resulting in unfair decision scenarios. Addressing bias in data
collection and interpretation is crucial to ensure the responsible integration of
SBDH and PGHD to improve patient outcomes and avoid potential disparities [226].

Translating SBDH data into meaningful results is a complex task, particularly in
the context of EHR incentive programmes. These programmes focus on capturing
data, optimizing the clinical workflow, and promoting continuous quality improvement to eliminate healthcare inequalities. The third stage emphasizes the importance of addressing the relationship between SBDH and health outcomes. Recent
research underscores the positive impact of incorporating SBDH into EHR, leading
to improved outcomes such as increased performance, higher medication adherence
rates, reduced hospitalization risk, and other positive indicators [231].

Furthermore, there are also barriers to the widespread implementation of SBDH
screening in healthcare encounters. Key SBDH measures are not routinely collected, and when collected, rarely validated instruments are employed, limiting the
secondary use of this valuable information. The obstacles include providers' unwill-
ingness to address patients' needs without clear resources, concerns about the
impact on patient–provider relationships, a lack of training, an absence of incentives
to record findings, and a lack of agreement on which SBDH to screen for and the
most reliable standardized tools [232].

Context challenges further complicate SBDH data collection, requiring special
considerations for sensitive situations. Factors such as unstable housing situations

when caring for a child or an elder or when dealing with a drug-dependent family member introduce complexities in the selection of appropriate scenarios and types of questions for each patient. Similar to the approach of patient-centred and personalized care, SBDH data collection practices need to be tailored for each patient scenario, whether conducted in person or via data collection technologies [228]. In navigating these challenges, the responsible and ethical use of SBDH data becomes imperative for fostering equitable healthcare practices and outcomes.

1.9.3   SBDH: Examples of Reuse

The Use of SBDH in Disease Prediction

The secondary use of SBDH data has demonstrated its potential in various impactful applications. Prediction models have been developed to identify patients at risk on the basis of socioeconomic factors. Research has shown that low socioeconomic status and socioeconomic distress are associated with the risk of comorbid substance use disorders and opioid misuse [233, 234]. Furthermore, studies have explored the use of SBDH in predicting suicide risk, with factors such as education level, employment status, and income significantly correlated with suicidal behaviour in mentally ill patients [235–237]. Tools such as the OxMIS have been designed to predict suicide in severely mentally ill patients, incorporating SBDH factors such as education and substance abuse [238].

The Use of SBDH in Disease Management

SBDH data integration has also proven valuable in designing interventions for improved disease management. Semantic extract, transform, and load (ETL) services and dashboard systems such as the MOSAIC have contributed to better managing conditions such as obesity and diabetes. For example, patient education on lifestyle interventions associated with improved glycaemic control in diabetes patients highlights the potential for the use of SBDH data to enhance disease management [239–241].

The Use of SBDH in the Prediction of Disease Progress and Outcome

Moreover, the reuse of SBDH data plays a pivotal role in predicting the progression and outcomes of various disease states. Factors such as housing status, including homelessness, and geographic location have been identified as influencing mental, behavioural, and neurodevelopmental disorders, as well as circulatory system diseases [242]. Geographic location, which acts as a surrogate for socioeconomic characteristics, has been associated with multiple diseases, health conditions, and high mortality rates [243]. These examples underscore the versatility and significance of SBDH data in informing healthcare decision-making, designing interventions, and predicting health outcomes.

The Use of SBDH in Improving the Design of Risk-Adjusted Payment Models and Performance-Based Incentives

The first US payment model, which includes SDBH variables, was described previously [230]. In October 2016, MassHealth, which includes Massachusetts' Medicaid and Children's Health Insurance programmes, added two SDBH variables: the neighbourhood stress score and the amount of unstable housing. Adding the available SDBH and other data (e.g. whether subjects used the services of the Departments of Mental Health or Developmental Services) to the diagnosis-based model led to improved matching of payments to costs for several vulnerable member categories. However, improving such SDBH risk adjustment models requires fairly complete information on SDBH factors in medical encounters and claims data, which is a problem noted by Torres and colleagues [228].

References

1. FDA (2023) Real-world evidence. https://www.fda.gov/science-research/science-and-research-special-topics/real-world-evidence. Accessed 25 June 2024
2. National Institute for Health and Care Excellence (NICE) (2024) Glossary. https://www.nice.org.uk/Glossary?letter=R#Real-world%20evidence. Accessed 25 June 2024
3. Liu F, Demosthenes P (2022) Real-world data: a brief review of the methods, applications, challenges and opportunities. BMC Med Res Methodol 22:287. https://doi.org/10.1186/S12874-022-01768-6
4. European Medicines Agency (2023) RWE_framework_to_support_EU_regulatory_decision_making_1688023939.pdf. Open Science Framework
5. Dang A (2023) Real-world evidence: a primer. Pharmaceut Med 37:25–36. https://doi.org/10.1007/s40290-022-00456-6
6. Dang A, Jagan Mohan Venkateswara Rao P, Kishore R, Vallish BN (2021) Real world safety of bevacizumab in cancer patients: a systematic literature review of case reports. Int J Risk Saf Med 32:163–173. https://doi.org/10.3233/JRS-194051
7. MarksMan Healthcare (2018) How RWE can impact clinical trial design and help in decision making? https://marksmanhealthcare.com/2018/10/24/how-rwe-can-impact-clinical-trial-design-and-help-in-decision-making/. Accessed 8 Nov 2023
8. Hernández MA, Stolfo SJ (1998) Real-world data is dirty: data cleansing and the merge/purge problem. Data Min Knowl Discov 2:9–37. https://doi.org/10.1023/A:1009761603038/METRICS
9. Corrigan-Curay J, Sacks L, Woodcock J (2018) Real-world evidence and real-world data for evaluating drug safety and effectiveness. JAMA 320:867–868. https://doi.org/10.1001/JAMA.2018.10136
10. Makady A, de Boer A, Hillege H et al (2017) What is real-world data? A review of definitions based on literature and stakeholder interviews. Value Health 20:858–865. https://doi.org/10.1016/J.JVAL.2017.03.008
11. Franklin JM, Schneeweiss S (2017) When and how can real world data analyses substitute for randomized controlled trials? Clin Pharmacol Ther 102:924–933. https://doi.org/10.1002/CPT.857
12. Djurisic S, Rath A, Gaber S et al (2017) Barriers to the conduct of randomized clinical trials within all disease areas. Trials 18:360. https://doi.org/10.1186/s13063-017-2099-9
13. Rudrapatna VA, Butte AJ (2020) Opportunities and challenges in using real-world data for health care. J Clin Invest 130:565–574. https://doi.org/10.1172/JCI129197

14. US Food & Drug Administration (2017) New drug therapy approvals 2017. https://www.academia.edu/36341647/New_Drug_Therapy_Approvals_2017_FDA_report. Accessed 8 Nov 2023

15. Chatterjee A, Chilukuri S, Fleming E, et al (2018) Real-world evidence: driving a new drug-development paradigm in oncology | McKinsey. https://www.mckinsey.com/industries/life-sciences/our-insights/real-world-evidence-driving-a-new-drug-development-paradigm-in-oncology. Accessed 8 Nov 2023

16. Li G, Sajobi TT, Menon BK et al (2016) Registry-based randomized controlled trials- what are the advantages, challenges, and areas for future research? J Clin Epidemiol 80:16–24. https://doi.org/10.1016/j.jclinepi.2016.08.003

17. Purpura CA, Garry EM, Honig N et al (2022) The role of real-world evidence in FDA-approved new drug and biologics licence applications. Clin Pharmacol Ther 111:135–144. https://doi.org/10.1002/CPT.2474

18. US Food & Drug Administration (2018) Framework for FDA's real-world evidence program. https://www.fda.gov/media/120060/download. Accessed 12 Nov 2023

19. DARWIN EU (2023) Data analysis and real world interrogation network. https://darwin-eu.org/. Accessed 11 Nov 2023

20. Harbaugh CM, Cooper JN (2018) Administrative databases. Semin Pediatr Surg 27:353–360. https://doi.org/10.1053/J.SEMPEDSURG.2018.10.001

21. Sutherland SM (2020) Big data and pediatric acute kidney injury: the promise of electronic health record systems. Front Pediatr 7:536. https://doi.org/10.3389/FPED.2019.00536

22. Gavrielov-Yusim N, Friger M (2014) Use of administrative medical databases in population-based research. J Epidemiol Community Health 68:283–287. https://doi.org/10.1136/JECH-2013-202744

23. Ulrich EH, So G, Zappitelli M, Chanchlani R (2021) A review on the application and limitations of administrative health care data for the study of acute kidney injury epidemiology and outcomes in children. Front Pediatr 9:742888. https://doi.org/10.3389/fped.2021.742888

24. Shrestha S, Dave AJ, Losina E, Katz JN (2016) Diagnostic accuracy of administrative data algorithms in the diagnosis of osteoarthritis: a systematic review. BMC Med Inform Decis Mak 16:82. https://doi.org/10.1186/S12911-016-0319-Y

25. Mazzali C, Maistriello M, Ieva F, Barbieri P (2015) Methodological issues in the use of administrative databases to study heart failure. In: Paganoni AM, Secchi P (eds) Advances in complex data modelling and computational methods in statistics, Contributions to statistics. Springer, pp 149–160

26. Parker SL, McGirt MJ (2015) Editorial: administrative database research. J Neurosurg 122:441–442. https://doi.org/10.3171/2014.4.JNS14689

27. Zarrinkoub R, Wettermark B, Wändell P et al (2013) The epidemiology of heart failure, based on data for 2.1 million inhabitants in Sweden. Eur J Heart Fail 15:995–1002. https://doi.org/10.1093/EURJHF/HFT064

28. Lipscombe LL, Hux JE (2007) Trends in diabetes incidence, incidence, and mortality in Ontario, Canada 1995-2005: a population-based study. Lancet 369:750–756. https://doi.org/10.1016/S0140-6736(07)60361-4

29. Koopman C, Bots ML, Van Oeffelen AAM et al (2013) Population trends and inequalities in incidence and short-term outcome of acute myocardial infarction between 1998 and 2007. Int J Cardiol 168:993–998. https://doi.org/10.1016/J.IJCARD.2012.10.036

30. Mazzali C, Duca P (2015) Use of administrative data in healthcare research. Intern Emerg Med 10:517–524. https://doi.org/10.1007/S11739-015-1213-9

31. Gao J, Moran E, Li YF, Almenoff PL (2014) Predicting potentially avoidable hospitalizations. Med Care 52:164–171. https://doi.org/10.1097/MLR.0000000000000041

32. Miguel A, Marques B, Freitas A et al (2013) Detection of adverse drug reactions using hospital databases-a nationwide study in Portugal. Pharmacoepidemiol Drug Saf 22:907–913. https://doi.org/10.1002/PDS.3468

33. Loft S, Poulsen HE (1996) Cancer risk and oxidative DNA damage in man. J Mol Med (Berl) 74:297–312. https://doi.org/10.1007/BF00207507

34. Annaratone L, De Palma G, Bonizzi G et al (2021) Basic principles of biobanking: from biological samples to precision medicine for patients. Virchows Arch 479:233. https://doi.org/10.1007/S00428-021-03151-0

35. Hewitt R, Watson P (2013) Defining biobank. Biopreserv Biobank 11:309–315. https://doi.org/10.1089/BIO.2013.0042

36. Ballantyne A (2019) Adjusting the focus: a public health ethics approach to data research. Bioethics 33:357–366. https://doi.org/10.1111/BIOE.12551

37. Harris JR, Burton P, Knoppers BM et al (2012) Toward a roadmap in global biobanking for health. Eur J Hum Genet 20:1105–1111. https://doi.org/10.1038/EJHG.2012.96

38. Jacobs G, Wolf A, Krawczak M, Lieb W (2018) Biobanks in the era of digital medicine. Clin Pharmacol Ther 103:761–762. https://doi.org/10.1002/CPT.968

39. Dhai A (2016) The WMA declaration of Taipei: human databases and biobanks for the common good. S Afr J Bioeth Law 9:50–51. https://doi.org/10.7196/SAJBL.2016.v9i2.270

40. Small AM, O'Donnell CJ, Damrauer SM (2018) Large-scale genomic biobanks and cardiovascular disease. Curr Cardiol Rep 20. https://doi.org/10.1007/S11886-018-0969-8

41. Gaziano JM, Concato J, Brophy M et al (2016) Million veteran program: a mega-biobank to study genetic influences on health and disease. J Clin Epidemiol 70:214–223. https://doi.org/10.1016/J.JCLINEPI.2015.09.016

42. Celis-Morales CA, Lyall DM, Welsh P et al (2017) Association between active commuting and incident cardiovascular disease, cancer, and mortality: prospective cohort study. BMJ 357:j1456. https://doi.org/10.1136/bmj.j1456

43. National Center for Advancing Translational Sciences (2024) Rare Diseases Clinical Research Network (RDCRN). https://ncats.nih.gov/research/research-activities/rdcrn. Accessed 25 June 2024

44. Genomics England (2024) 100,000 genomes project. https://www.genomicsengland.co.uk/initiatives/100000-genomes-project. Accessed 25 June 2024

45. Kalia SS, Adelman K, Bale SJ et al (2017) Recommendations for reporting of secondary findings in clinical exome and genome sequencing, 2016 update (ACMG SF v2.0): a policy statement of the American College of Medical Genetics and Genomics. Genet Med 19:249–255. https://doi.org/10.1038/GIM.2016.190

46. Harris J, Sulston J (2004) Genetic equity. Nat Rev Genet 5:796–800. https://doi.org/10.1038/NRG1454

47. Editorial (2021) Precision medicine needs an equity agenda. Nat Med 27:737. https://doi.org/10.1038/S41591-021-01373-Y

48. Rotimi C, Abayomi A, Abimiku A et al (2014) Enabling the genomic revolution in Africa: H3Africa is developing capacity for health-related genomics research in Africa. Science 344:1346. https://doi.org/10.1126/SCIENCE.1251546

49. Wall JD, Stawiski EW, Ratan A et al (2019) The GenomeAsia 100K project enables genetic discoveries across Asia. Nature 576:106–111. https://doi.org/10.1038/S41586-019-1793-Z

50. Robine N, Varmus H (2022) New York's Polyethnic-1000: a regional initiative to understand how diverse ancestries influence the risk, progression, and treatment of cancers. Trends Cancer 8:269–272. https://doi.org/10.1016/J.TRECAN.2021.11.005

51. Gange SJ, Golub ET (2016) From smallpox to big data: the next 100 years of epidemiologic methods. Am J Epidemiol 183:423–426. https://doi.org/10.1093/AJE/KWV150

52. Ehrenstein V, Nielsen H, Pedersen AB et al (2017) Clinical epidemiology in the era of big data: new opportunities, familiar challenges. Clin Epidemiol 9:245–250. https://doi.org/10.2147/CLEP.S129779

53. Sanderson SC, Brothers KB, Mercaldo ND et al (2017) Public attitudes toward consent and data sharing in biobank research: a large multisite experimental survey in the US. Am J Hum Genet 100:414–427. https://doi.org/10.1016/J.AJHG.2017.01.021

54. D'Abramo F, Schildmann J, Vollmann J (2015) Research participants' perceptions and views on consent for biobank research: a review of empirical data and ethical analysis. BMC Med Ethics 16:60. https://doi.org/10.1186/S12910-015-0053-5

55. Coppola L, Cianflone A, Grimaldi AM et al (2019) Biobanking in health care: evolution and future directions. J Transl Med 17:172. https://doi.org/10.1186/S12967-019-1922-3

56. Boeckhout M, Zielhuis GA, Bredenoord AL (2018) The FAIR guiding principles for data stewardship: fair enough? Eur J Hum Genet 26:931–936. https://doi.org/10.1038/S41431-018-0160-0

57. Holub P, Kohlmayer F, Prasser F et al (2018) Enhancing reuse of data and biological material in medical research: from FAIR to FAIR-health. Biopreserv Biobank 16:97. https://doi.org/10.1089/BIO.2017.0110

58. Ranasinghe S, Pichler H, Eder J (2018) Report on data quality in biobanks: problems, issues, state-of-the-art. https://doi.org/10.48550/arXiv.1812.10423

59. Kodra Y, Weinbach J, Posada-De-La-Paz M et al (2018) Recommendations for improving the quality of rare disease registries. Int J Environ Res Public Health 15. https://doi.org/10.3390/IJERPH15081644

60. Moore HM, Compton CC, Alper J, Vaught JB (2011) International approaches to advancing biospecimen science. Cancer Epidemiol Biomarkers Prev 20:729. https://doi.org/10.1158/1055-9965.EPI-11-0021

61. OECD (2007) OECD best practice guidelines for biological resource centres. https://www.oecd.org/health/biotech/oecdbestpracticeguidelinesforbiologicalresourcecentres.htm. Accessed 26 June 2024

62. Campbell LD, Astrin JJ, DeSouza Y et al (2018) The 2018 revision of the ISBER best practices: summary of changes and the editorial team's development process. Biopreserv Biobank 16:3. https://doi.org/10.1089/BIO.2018.0001

63. National Cancer Institute (2016) NCI best practices for biospecimen resources

64. Mendy M, Caboux E, Lawlor RT et al (2017) Common minimum technical standards and protocols for biobanks dedicated to cancer research. International Agency for Research on Cancer

65. Council for International Organizations of Medical Sciences (CIOMS) in collaboration with the World Health Organization (WHO) (2016) International ethical guidelines for health-related research involving humans. www.cioms.ch. Accessed 26 June 2024

66. Nuffield Council on Bioethics (2015) The collection, linking and use of data in biomedical research and health care: ethical issues. A guide to the report. Accessed 26 June 2024

67. Recommendations of the European Society of Human Genetics (2003) Data storage and DNA banking for biomedical research: technical, social and ethical issues. Eur J Hum Genet 11:S8–S10. https://doi.org/10.1038/sj.ejhg.5201115

68. ISO (2018) ISO 20387:2018 - biotechnology — biobanking — general requirements for biobanking. https://www.iso.org/standard/67888.html. Accessed 26 June 2024

69. Conroy MC, Lacey B, Bešević J et al (2023) UK biobank: a globally important resource for cancer research. Br J Cancer 128:519–527. https://doi.org/10.1038/S41416-022-02053-5

70. Conroy M, Sellors J, Effingham M et al (2019) The advantages of UK Biobank's open-access strategy for health research. J Intern Med 286:389–397. https://doi.org/10.1111/JOIM.12955

71. Chadeau-Hyam M, Bodinier B, Elliott J et al (2020) Risk factors for positive and negative COVID-19 tests: a cautious and in-depth analysis of UK biobank data. Int J Epidemiol 49:1454–1467. https://doi.org/10.1093/IJE/DYAA134

72. Statistics Canada Biobank. https://www.statcan.gc.ca/en/microdata/biobank. Accessed 11 Nov 2023

73. Chen Z, Chen J, Collins R et al (2011) China Kadoorie Biobank of 0.5 million people: survey methods, baseline characteristics and long-term follow-up. Int J Epidemiol 40:1652–1666. https://doi.org/10.1093/IJE/DYR120

74. China Kadoorie Biobank (CKB). https://www.ckbiobank.org/. Accessed 11 Nov 2023

75. Nagai A, Hirata M, Kamatani Y et al (2017) Overview of the BioBank Japan project: study design and profile. J Epidemiol 27:S2–S8. https://doi.org/10.1016/J.JE.2016.12.005
76. BioBank Japan. https://biobankjp.org/en/index.html. Accessed 11 Nov 2023
77. Alver M, Palover M, Saar A et al (2019) Recall by genotype and cascade screening for familial hypercholesterolemia in a population-based biobank from Estonia. Genet Med 21:1173–1180. https://doi.org/10.1038/S41436-018-0311-2
78. Estonian Biobank. https://genomics.ut.ee/en/content/estonian-biobank. Accessed 11 Nov 2023
79. World Health Organization. Clinical trials. https://www.who.int/health-topics/clinical-trials/#tab=tab_1. Accessed 9 Nov 2023
80. NIH Grants & Funding NIH's. Definition of a clinical trial. https://grants.nih.gov/policy/clinical-trials/definition.htm. Accessed 26 June 2024
81. European Medicines Agency (2024) Clinical trials information system (CTIS): online training modules. https://www.ema.europa.eu/en/human-regulatory-overview/research-development/clinical-trials-human-medicines/clinical-trials-information-system-training-support/clinical-trials-information-system-ctis-online-training-modules. Accessed 26 June 2024
82. U.S. Food & Drug Administration (FDA) (2020) FDA continues to support transparency and collaboration in drug approval process as the clinical data summary pilot concludes. https://www.fda.gov/news-events/press-announcements/fda-continues-support-transparency-and-collaboration-drug-approval-process-clinical-data-summary. Accessed 26 June 2024
83. National Institutes of Health (NIH) (2022) NIH office of data science strategy announces new initiative to improve access to NIH-funded data. https://datascience.nih.gov/news/nih-office-of-data-science-strategy-announces-new-initiative-to-improve-data-access. Accessed 26 June 2024
84. Research Councils UK (2015) Guidance on best practice in the management of research data. http://www.oecd.org/sti/sci-tech/38500813.pdf. Accessed 26 June 2024
85. Ohmann C, Banzi R, Canham S et al (2017) Sharing and reuse of individual participant data from clinical trials: principles and recommendations. BMJ Open 7:18647. https://doi.org/10.1136/bmjopen-2017-018647
86. Medical Research Council (MRC) (2016) MRC policy on open research data from clinical trials and public health intervention studies. https://www.ukri.org/wp-content/uploads/2021/08/MRC-0208212-20200116_MRC-Policy-on-Open-Research-Data_FINAL-update.pdf. Accessed 12 Nov 2023
87. Miron L, Gonçalves RS, Musen MA (2020) Obstacles to the reuse of study metadata in ClinicalTrials.gov. Sci Data 7:443. https://doi.org/10.1038/S41597-020-00780-Z
88. Committee on Strategies for Responsible Sharing of Clinical Trial Data; Board on Health Sciences Policy; Institute of Medicine (2015) Guiding principles for sharing clinical trial data. National Academies Press (US)
89. Chan A-W, Song F, Vickers A et al (2014) Increasing value and reducing waste: addressing inaccessible research. Lancet 383:257–266. https://doi.org/10.1016/S0140-6736(13)62296-5
90. EFPIA, Barnes B (2019) Safeguards framework for secondary use of clinical trial data for scientific research. https://www.efpia.eu/media/413227/position-paper-safeguards-framework-for-secondary-use-of-clinical-trial-data-for-scientific-research-September-2019.pdf. Accessed 26 June 2024
91. Wilkinson T, Sinha S, Peek N, Geifman N (2019) Clinical trial data reuse—overcoming complexities in trial design and data sharing. Trials 20:513. https://doi.org/10.1186/s13063-019-3627-6
92. Wilkinson T, Sinha S, Peek N, Geifman N (2019) Clinical trial data reuse - overcoming complexities in trial design and data sharing. Trials 20:513. https://doi.org/10.1186/S13063-019-3627-6/FIGURES/1
93. O'Connor CM, van Veldhuisen DJ (2017) Data sharing from the editors' perspective. JACC Heart Fail 5:314–315. https://doi.org/10.1016/j.jchf.2017.02.007

94. Geifman N, Kennedy RE, Schneider LS et al (2018) Data-driven identification of endophe-notypes of Alzheimer's disease progression: implications for clinical trials and therapeutic interventions. Alzheimers Res Ther 10:4. https://doi.org/10.1186/S13195-017-0332-0

95. Hill-McManus D, Hughes DA (2021) Combining model-based clinical trial simulation, phar-macoeconomics, and value of information to optimize trial design. CPT Pharmacometrics Syst Pharmacol 10:75–83. https://doi.org/10.1002/PSP4.12579

96. Nissen SE, Wolski K (2007) Effect of rosiglitazone on the risk of myocardial infarction and death from cardiovascular causes. N Engl J Med 356:2457–2471. https://doi.org/10.1056/NEJMOA072761

97. Fujiwara Y, Horita N, Adib E et al (2024) Treatment-related adverse events, including fatal toxicities, in patients with solid tumours receiving neoadjuvant and adjuvant immune check-point blockade: a systematic review and meta-analysis of randomized controlled trials. Lancet Oncol 25:62–75. https://doi.org/10.1016/S1470-2045(23)00524-7

98. Ambinder EP (2005) Electronic health records. J Oncol Pract 1:57–63. https://doi.org/10.1200/JOP.2005.1.2.57

99. Shah SM, Khan RA (2020) Secondary use of electronic health record: opportunities and chal-lenges. IEEE Access 8:136947–136965. https://doi.org/10.1109/ACCESS.2020.3011099

100. Gianfrancesco MA, Goldstein ND (2021) A narrative review on the validity of electronic health record-based research in epidemiology. BMC Med Res Methodol 21:234. https://doi.org/10.1186/S12874-021-01416-5

101. Chaudhry B, Wang J, Wu S et al (2006) Systematic review: impact of health information technology on quality, efficiency, and costs of medical care. Ann Intern Med 144:742–752. https://doi.org/10.7326/0003-4819-144-10-200605160-00125

102. Sandhu E, Weinstein S, McKethan A, Jain SH (2012) Secondary uses of electronic health record data: benefits and barriers. Jt Comm J Qual Patient Saf 38:34–40. https://doi.org/10.1016/S1553-7250(12)38005-7

103. DiMasi JA, Hansen RW, Grabowski HG (2003) The price of innovation: new esti-mates of drug development costs. J Health Econ 22:151–185. https://doi.org/10.1016/S0167-6296(02)00126-1

104. Elkin PL, Trusko BE, Koppel R et al (2010) Secondary use of clinical data. Stud Health Technol Inform 155:14–29

105. Yim W-W, Wheeler AJ, Curtin C et al (2018) Secondary use of electronic medical records for clinical research: challenges and opportunities. Converg Sci Phys Oncol 4:014001. https://doi.org/10.1088/2057-1739/AAA905

106. European Commission (2024) European health data space. https://health.ec.europa.eu/ehealth-digital-health-and-care/european-health-data-space_en. Accessed 12 Jan 2024

107. Coorevits P, Sundgren M, Klein GO et al (2013) Electronic health records: new opportunities for clinical research. J Intern Med 274:547–560. https://doi.org/10.1111/joim.12119

108. Xiao Y, Wu J, Lin Z, Zhao X (2018) A deep learning-based multimodel ensemble method for cancer prediction. Comput Methods Prog Biomed 153:1–9. https://doi.org/10.1016/J.CMPB.2017.09.005

109. Willyard C (2017) The drug-resistant bacteria that pose the greatest health threats. Nature 543:15. https://doi.org/10.1038/NATURE.2017.21550

110. Spicknall IH, Looker KJ, Gottlieb SL et al (2019) Review of mathematical models of HSV-2 vaccination: implications for vaccine development. Vaccine 37:7396–7407. https://doi.org/10.1016/J.VACCINE.2018.02.067

111. Shuey MM, Lee KM, Keaton J et al (2023) A genetically supported drug repurposing pipeline for diabetes treatment using electronic health records. EBioMedicine 94:104674. https://doi.org/10.1016/J.EBIOM.2023.104674

112. Lanzillotta-Rangeley J, Clark A, Christianson A, Kalarchian MA (2020) Association of prescription opioid exposure and patient factors with prolonged postoperative opioid use in opioid-Naïve patients. AANA J 88:18–26

113. Atreja A, Gordon SM, Pollock DA et al (2008) Opportunities and challenges in utilizing electronic health records for infection surveillance, prevention, and control. Am J Infect Control 36:S37–S46. https://doi.org/10.1016/J.AJIC.2008.01.002

114. Keck JW, Redd JT, Cheek JE et al (2014) Influenza surveillance using electronic health records in the American Indian and Alaska native population. J Am Med Inform Assoc 21:132–138. https://doi.org/10.1136/AMIAJNL-2012-001591

115. Odero W, Rotich J, Yiannoutsos CT et al (2007) Innovative approaches to application of information technology in disease surveillance and prevention in Western Kenya. J Biomed Inform 40:390–397. https://doi.org/10.1016/J.JBI.2006.12.007

116. Loonsk JW (2004) BioSense--a national initiative for early detection and quantification of public health emergencies. MMWR Suppl 53:53–55

117. Kapoor A, Guha S, Kanti Das M et al (2020) Digital healthcare: the only solution for better healthcare during COVID-19 pandemic? Indian Heart J 72:61–64. https://doi.org/10.1016/J.IHJ.2020.04.001

118. Esposito P, Dal Canton A (2014) Clinical audit, a valuable tool to improve quality of care: general methodology and applications in nephrology. World J Nephrol 3:249. https://doi.org/10.5527/WJN.V3.I4.249

119. Litzelman DK, Dittus RS, Miller ME, Tierney WM (1993) Requiring physicians to respond to computerized reminders improves their compliance with preventive care protocols. J Gen Intern Med 8:311–317. https://doi.org/10.1007/BF02600144

120. Kucher N, Koo S, Quiroz R et al (2005) Electronic alerts to prevent venous thromboembolism among hospitalized patients. N Engl J Med 352:969–977. https://doi.org/10.1056/NEJMoa041533

121. CMS (2011) Medicare physician group practice demonstration. https://www.cms.gov/priorities/innovation/innovation-models/medicare-demonstrations/medicare-physician-group-practice-demonstration. Accessed 26 June 2024

122. Lee TH, Bothe A, Steele GD (2012) How Geisinger structures its physicians' compensation to support improvements in quality, efficiency, and volume. Health Aff (Millwood) 31:2068–2073. https://doi.org/10.1377/HLTHAFF.2011.0940

123. Paulus RA (2009) ProvenCare: Geisinger's model for care transformation through innovative clinical initiatives and value creation. Am Health Drug Benefits 2:122–127

124. Rung J, Brazma A (2013) Reuse of public genome-wide gene expression data. Nat Rev Genet 14:89–99. https://doi.org/10.1038/NRG3394

125. Domon B, Aebersold R (2006) Mass spectrometry and protein analysis. Science 312:212–217. https://doi.org/10.1126/SCIENCE.1124619

126. Tezel G (2013) A proteomics view of the molecular mechanisms and biomarkers of glaucomatous neurodegeneration. Prog Retin Eye Res 35:18–43. https://doi.org/10.1016/J.PRETEYERES.2013.01.004

127. FDA, CDER, CDRH, CBER (2018) E18 genomic sampling and management of genomic data guidance for industry. https://www.fda.gov/files/drugs/published/E18-Genomic-Sampling-and-Management-of-Genomic-Data-Guidance-for-Industry.pdf. Accessed 26 June 2024

128. McCarty CA, Chisholm RL, Chute CG et al (2011) The eMERGE network: a consortium of biorepositories linked to electronic medical records data for conducting genomic studies. BMC Med Genet 4:13. https://doi.org/10.1186/1755-8794-4-13

129. European Commission (2024) Shaping Europe's digital future. European "1+ Million Genomes" Initiative. https://digital-strategy.ec.europa.eu/en/policies/1million-genomes. Accessed 1 Oct 2024

130. Tenopir C, Rice NM, Allard S et al (2020) Data sharing, management, use, and reuse: practices and perceptions of scientists worldwide. PLoS One 15:e0229003. https://doi.org/10.1371/JOURNAL.PONE.0229003

131. Curty RG, Crowston K, Specht A et al (2017) Attitudes and norms affecting scientists' data reuse. PLoS One 12:e0189288. https://doi.org/10.1371/JOURNAL.PONE.0189288

132. Subramanian SL, Kitchen RR, Alexander R et al (2015) Integration of extracellular RNA profiling data using metadata, biomedical ontologies and linked data technologies. J Extracell Vesicles 4:27497. https://doi.org/10.3402/JEV.V4.27497

133. Wade TD (2014) Refining gold from existing data. Curr Opin Allergy Clin Immunol 14:181–185. https://doi.org/10.1097/ACI.0000000000000051

134. Safran C (2017) Update on data reuse in health care. Yearb Med Inform 26:24–27. https://doi.org/10.15265/IY-2017-013

135. Raju HB, Tsinoremas NF, Capobianco E (2016) Emerging putative associations between non-coding RNAs and protein-coding genes in neuropathic pain: added value from reusing microarray data. Front Neurol 7:168. https://doi.org/10.3389/FNEUR.2016.00168

136. McKiernan EC, Bourne PE, Brown CT et al (2016) How open science helps researchers succeed. Elife 5:e16800. https://doi.org/10.7554/ELIFE.16800

137. Leitner F, Bielza C, Hill SL, Larrañaga P (2016) Data publications correlate with citation impact. Front Neurosci 10:419. https://doi.org/10.3389/FNINS.2016.00419

138. Ali-Khan SE, Harris LW, Gold ER (2017) Motivating participation in open science by examining researcher incentives. Elife 6:e29319. https://doi.org/10.7554/ELIFE.29319

139. NCBI Resource Coordinators (2017) Database resources of the National Center for Biotechnology Information NCBI Resource Coordinators. Nucleic Acids Res 45:D12–D17. https://doi.org/10.1093/nar/gkw1071

140. Sayers EW, Cavanaugh M, Clark K et al (2019) GenBank. Nucleic Acids Res 47:D94–D99. https://doi.org/10.1093/nar/gky989

141. Sayers EW, Agarwala R, Bolton EE et al (2019) Database resources of the National Center for Biotechnology Information. Nucleic Acids Res 47:D23–D28. https://doi.org/10.1093/nar/gky1069

142. Perez-Riverol Y, Alpi E, Wang R et al (2015) Making proteomics data accessible and reusable: current state of proteomics databases and repositories. Proteomics 15:930–949. https://doi.org/10.1002/PMIC.201400302

143. Gostev M, Faulconbridge A, Brandizi M et al (2012) The BioSample Database (BioSD) at the European Bioinformatics Institute. Nucleic Acids Res 40:D64–D70. https://doi.org/10.1093/NAR/GKR937

144. Altelaar AFM, Munoz J, Heck AJR (2013) Next-generation proteomics: towards an integrative view of proteome dynamics. Nat Rev Genet 14:35–48. https://doi.org/10.1038/NRG3356

145. Distler U, Kuharev J, Navarro P et al (2014) Drift time-specific collision energies enable deep-coverage data-independent acquisition proteomics. Nat Methods 11:167–170. https://doi.org/10.1038/NMETH.2767

146. Lanucara F, Holman SW, Gray CJ, Eyers CE (2014) The power of ion mobility-mass spectrometry for structural characterization and the study of conformational dynamics. Nat Chem 6:281–294. https://doi.org/10.1038/NCHEM.1889

147. Riffle M, Eng JK (2009) Proteomics data repositories. Proteomics 9:4653–4663. https://doi.org/10.1002/PMIC.200900216

148. Craig R, Cortens JP, Beavis RC (2004) Open source system for analysing, validating, and storing protein identification data. J Proteome Res 3:1234–1242. https://doi.org/10.1021/PR049882H

149. Farrah T, Deutsch EW, Omenn GS et al (2014) The state of the human proteome in 2013 as viewed through PeptideAtlas: comparing the kidney, urine, and plasma proteomes for the biology and disease-driven human proteome project. J Proteome Res 13:60–75. https://doi.org/10.1021/PR4010037

150. Vizcaíno JA, Côté RG, Csordas A et al (2013) The PRoteomics IDEntifications (PRIDE) database and associated tools: status in 2013. Nucleic Acids Res 41. https://doi.org/10.1093/NAR/GKS1262

151. Slotta DJ, Barrett T, Edgar R (2009) NCBI peptidome: a new public repository for mass spectrometry peptide identifications. Nat Biotechnol 27:600–601. https://doi.org/10.1038/NBT0709-600

152. Smith BE, Hill JA, Gjukich MA, Andrews PC (2011) Tranche distributed repository and ProteomeCommons.org. Methods Mol Biol 696:123–145. https://doi.org/10.1007/978-1-60761-987-1_8

153. Ezkurdia I, Vázquez J, Valencia A, Tress M (2014) Analysing the first drafts of the human proteome. J Proteome Res 13:3854. https://doi.org/10.1021/PR500572Z

154. Kohane IS, Valtchinov VI (2012) Quantifying the white blood cell transcriptome as an accessible window to the multiorgan transcriptome. Bioinformatics 28:538–545. https://doi.org/10.1093/BIOINFORMATICS/BTR713

155. Lukk M, Kapushesky M, Nikkilä J et al (2010) A global map of human gene expression. Nat Biotechnol 28:322–324. https://doi.org/10.1038/nbt0410-322

156. Ojala KA, Kilpinen SK, Kallioniemi OP (2011) Classification of unknown primary tumors with a data-driven method based on a large microarray reference database. Genome Med 3:63. https://doi.org/10.1186/GM279

157. Tseng GC, Ghosh D, Feingold E (2012) Comprehensive literature review and statistical considerations for microarray meta-analysis. Nucleic Acids Res 40:3785–3799. https://doi.org/10.1093/NAR/GKR1265

158. Kang DD, Sibille E, Kaminski N, Tseng GC (2012) MetaQC: objective quality control and inclusion/exclusion criteria for genomic meta-analysis. Nucleic Acids Res 40:e15. https://doi.org/10.1093/NAR/GKR1071

159. Ramasamy A, Mondry A, Holmes CC, Altman DG (2008) Key issues in conducting a meta-analysis of gene expression microarray datasets. PLoS Med 5:e184. https://doi.org/10.1371/JOURNAL.PMED.0050184

160. Vilardell M, Rasche A, Thormann A et al (2011) Meta-analysis of heterogeneous down syndrome data reveals consistent genome-wide dosage effects related to neurological processes. BMC Genomics 12:229. https://doi.org/10.1186/1471-2164-12-229

161. Chen M, Wang K, Zhang L et al (2011) The discovery of putative urine markers for the specific detection of prostate tumor by integrative mining of public genomic profiles. PLoS One 6:e28552. https://doi.org/10.1371/JOURNAL.PONE.0028552

162. Gundem G, Perez-Llamas C, Jene-Sanz A et al (2010) IntOGen: integration and data mining of multidimensional oncogenomic data. Nat Methods 7:92–93. https://doi.org/10.1038/NMETH0210-92

163. Halling-Brown MD, Bulusu KC, Patel M et al (2012) canSAR: an integrated cancer public translational research and drug discovery resource. Nucleic Acids Res 40:D947–D956. https://doi.org/10.1093/NAR/GKR881

164. Lamb J, Crawford ED, Peck D et al (2006) The connectivity map: using gene-expression signatures to connect small molecules, genes, and disease. Science 313:1929–1935. https://doi.org/10.1126/science.1132939

165. Brooke EM, WHO (1974) The current and future use of registers in health information systems. https://iris.who.int/handle/10665/36936. Accessed 26 June 2024

166. National Committee on Vital and Health Statistics (2022) Frequently asked questions about medical and public health registries What is a registry? https://ncvhs.hhs.gov/wp-content/uploads/2022/11/FAQ-on-Public-Health-Registries.pdf. Accessed 26 June 2024

167. National Program of Cancer Registries (NPCRs) | CDC. https://www.cdc.gov/cancer/npcr/index.htm. Accessed 11 Nov 2023

168. Hallstrom BR, Hughes RE, Huddleston JI (2022) State-based and National U.S. Registries: the Michigan Arthroplasty Registry Collaborative Quality Initiative (MARCQI), California Joint Replacement Registry (CJRR), and American Joint Replacement Registry (AJRR). J Bone Joint Surg Am 104:18–22. https://doi.org/10.2106/JBJS.22.00564

169. Choquet R, Landais P (2014) The French national registry for rare diseases: an integrated model from care to epidemiology and research. Orphanet J Rare Dis 9:O7. https://doi.org/10.1186/1750-1172-9-S1-O7

170. Newton J, Garner S, University of Oxford. Institute of Health Sciences (2002) Disease registers in England: a report commissioned by the Department of Health Policy Research programme in support of the White Paper entitled Saving lives: our healthier nation

171. Gliklich RE, Dreyer NA, Leavy MB (2014) Registries for evaluating patient outcomes: a user's guide, 3rd edn. AHRQ Methods for Effective Health Care, Rockville, MD

172. Schmidt M, Schmidt SAJ, Sandegaard JL et al (2015) The Danish National Patient Registry: a review of content, data quality, and research potential. Clin Epidemiol 7:449–490. https://doi.org/10.2147/CLEP.S91125

173. Pop B, Fetica B, Blaga ML et al (2019) The role of medical registries, potential applications and limitations. Med Pharm Rep 92:7–14. https://doi.org/10.15386/CJMED-1015

174. Levine MN, Julian JA (2016) Registries that show efficacy: good, but not good enough. J Clin Oncol 26(33):5316–5319. https://doi.org/10.1200/JCO.2008.18.3996

175. Awaya A, Kuroiwa Y (2020) The relationship between annual airborne pollen levels and occurrence of all cancers, and lung, stomach, colorectal, pancreatic and breast cancers: a retrospective study from the National Registry Database of Cancer Incidence in Japan, 1975-2015. Int J Environ Res Public Health 17:3950. https://doi.org/10.3390/IJERPH17113950

176. Dadonienė J, Charukevič G, Jasionytė G et al (2021) Mortality in inflammatory rheumatic diseases: Lithuanian National Registry Data and systematic review. Int J Environ Res Public Health 18:12338. https://doi.org/10.3390/IJERPH182312338

177. Harris IA, Kirwan DP, Peng Y et al (2022) Increased early mortality after total knee arthroplasty using conventional instrumentation compared with technology-assisted surgery: an analysis of linked national registry data. BMJ Open 12:e055859. https://doi.org/10.1136/BMJOPEN-2021-055859

178. Honkila M, Wikström E, Renko M et al (2017) Probability of vertical transmission of *Chlamydia trachomatis* estimated from national registry data. Sex Transm Infect 93:416–420. https://doi.org/10.1136/sextrans-2016-052884

179. Johnston DS (2017) Digital maturity: are we ready to use technology in the NHS? Future Healthc J 4:189–192. https://doi.org/10.7861/FUTUREHOSP.4-3-189

180. The National Cardiovascular Data Registry (2023) https://cvquality.acc.org/NCDR-Home. Accessed 11 Nov 2023

181. Kutcher MA, Klein LW, Ou FS et al (2009) Percutaneous coronary interventions in facilities without cardiac surgery on site: a report from the National Cardiovascular Data Registry (NCDR). J Am Coll Cardiol 54:16–24. https://doi.org/10.1016/J.JACC.2009.03.038

182. Cardona-Hernandez R, Schwandt A, Alkandari H et al (2021) Glycemic outcome associated with insulin pump and glucose sensor use in children and adolescents with type 1 diabetes. Data from the international pediatric registry SWEET. Diabetes Care 44:1176–1184. https://doi.org/10.2337/DC20-1674

183. Lanzinger S, Zimmermann A, Ranjan AG et al (2022) A collaborative comparison of international pediatric diabetes registries. Pediatr Diabetes 23:627–640. https://doi.org/10.1111/PEDI.13362

184. Van Dijk PCW, Jager KJ, Stengel B et al (2005) Renal replacement therapy for diabetic end-stage renal disease: data from 10 registries in Europe (1991-2000). Kidney Int 67:1489–1499. https://doi.org/10.1111/J.1523-1755.2005.00227.X

185. European Medicines Agency (2011) Committee for medicinal products for human use (CHMP) Guideline on the clinical investigation of recombinant and human plasma-derived factor VIII products. www.ema.europa.ee. Accessed 26 June 2024

186. Ali S, Kjeken R, Niederlaender C et al (2020) The European medicines agency review of Kymriah (Tisagenlecleucel) for the treatment of acute lymphoblastic leukemia and diffuse large B-cell lymphoma. Oncologist 25:e321–e327. https://doi.org/10.1634/THEONCOLOGIST.2019-0233

187. Papadouli I, Mueller-Berghaus J, Beuneu C et al (2020) EMA review of Axicabtagene Ciloleucel (Yescarta) for the treatment of diffuse large B-cell lymphoma. Oncologist 25:894–902. https://doi.org/10.1634/THEONCOLOGIST.2019-0646

188. Paper W, Shapiro M, Johnston D, et al (2012) Patient-generated health data white paper. Accessed 26 June 2024
189. Bourke A, Dixon WG, Roddam A et al (2020) Incorporating patient generated health data into pharmacoepidemiological research. Pharmacoepidemiol Drug Saf 29:1540–1549. https://doi.org/10.1002/PDS.5169
190. Codella J, Partovian C, Chang HY, Chen CH (2018) Data quality challenges for person-generated health and wellness data. IBM J Res Dev 62(1):1–3. https://doi.org/10.1147/JRD.2017.2762218
191. FDA, Office of the Commissioner (1998) Recruiting study subjects. https://www.fda.gov/regulatory-information/search-fda-guidance-documents/recruiting-study-subjects. Accessed 27 June 2024
192. Office of the National Coordinator for Health Information Technology (2018) Conceptualizing a data infrastructure for the capture, use, and sharing of patient-generated health data in care delivery and research through 2024. Accessed 27 June 2024
193. Jim HSL, Hoogland AI, Brownstein NC et al (2020) Innovations in research and clinical care using patient-generated health data. CA Cancer J Clin 70:182–199. https://doi.org/10.3322/CAAC.21608
194. Huang Y, Upadhyay U, Dhar E et al (2022) A scoping review to assess adherence to and clinical outcomes of wearable devices in the cancer population. Cancers (Basel) 14:4437. https://doi.org/10.3390/CANCERS14184437
195. Linwood SL (2022) Digital health. Exon Publications
196. Krist AH, Tong ST, Aycock RA, Longo DR (2017) Engaging patients in decision-making and behavior change to promote prevention. Inf Serv Use 37:105–122. https://doi.org/10.3233/ISU-170826
197. Abdolkhani R, Gray K, Borda A, DeSouza R (2019) Patient-generated health data management and quality challenges in remote patient monitoring. JAMIA Open 2:471–478. https://doi.org/10.1093/JAMIAOPEN/OOZ036
198. Health IT Buzz, DeSalvo KB, Samuel J (2016) Examining oversight of the privacy & security of health data collected by entities not regulated by HIPAA. https://www.healthit.gov/buzz-blog/privacy-and-security/examining-oversight-privacy-security-health-data-collected-entities-not-regulated-hipaa. Accessed 27 June 2024
199. European Commission (2018) Reform of EU data protection rules. https://commission.europa.eu/law/law-topic/data-protection/reform_en. Accessed 27 June 2024
200. FDA, OHRP, CDER, et al (2016) Use of electronic informed consent questions and answers guidance for institutional review boards, investigators, and sponsors. https://www.fda.gov/media/116850/download. Accessed 27 June 2024
201. Mooney KH, Beck SL, Friedman RH et al (2014) Automated monitoring of symptoms during ambulatory chemotherapy and oncology providers' use of the information: a randomized controlled clinical trial. Support Care Cancer 22:2343–2350. https://doi.org/10.1007/s00520-014-2216-1
202. Wheelock AE, Bock MA, Martin EL et al (2015) SIS.NET: a randomized controlled trial evaluating a web-based system for symptom management after treatment of breast cancer. Cancer 121:893–899. https://doi.org/10.1002/CNCR.29088
203. Kearney N, McCann L, Norrie J et al (2009) Evaluation of a mobile phone-based, advanced symptom management system (ASyMS) in the management of chemotherapy-related toxicity. Support Care Cancer 17:437–444. https://doi.org/10.1007/S00520-008-0515-0
204. Nelson BW, Allen NB (2019) Accuracy of consumer wearable heart rate measurement during an ecologically valid 24-hour period: intraindividual validation study. JMIR Mhealth Uhealth 7:e10828. https://doi.org/10.2196/10828
205. Thomson EA, Nuss K, Comstock A et al (2019) Heart rate measures from the Apple Watch, Fitbit Charge HR 2, and electrocardiogram across different exercise intensities. J Sports Sci 37:1411–1419. https://doi.org/10.1080/02640414.2018.1560644

206. Haberman ZC, Jahn RT, Bose R et al (2015) Wireless smartphone ECG enables large-scale screening in diverse populations. J Cardiovasc Electrophysiol 26:520–526. https://doi.org/10.1111/JCE.12634

207. Klesges RC, Klbsges LM, Swenson AM, Pheley AM (1985) A validation of two motion sensors in the prediction of child and adult physical activity levels. Am J Epidemiol 122:400–410. https://doi.org/10.1093/OXFORDJOURNALS.AJE.A114121

208. Breteler MJM, Janssen JH, Spiering W et al (2019) Measuring free-living physical activity with three commercially available activity monitors for telemonitoring purposes: validation study. JMIR Form Res 3:e11489. https://doi.org/10.2196/11489

209. Zhang P, Godin SD, Owens MV (2019) Measuring the validity and reliability of the Apple Watch as a physical activity monitor. J Sports Med Phys Fitness 59:784–790. https://doi.org/10.23736/S0022-4707.18.08339-1

210. Bai Y, Hibbing P, Mantis C, Welk GJ (2018) Comparative evaluation of heart rate-based monitors: Apple Watch vs Fitbit charge HR. J Sports Sci 36:1734–1741. https://doi.org/10.1080/02640414.2017.1412235

211. Nolan M, Mitchell JR, Doyle-Baker PK (2014) Validity of the Apple iPhone®/iPod Touch® as an accelerometer-based physical activity monitor: a proof-of-concept study. J Phys Act Health 11:759–769. https://doi.org/10.1123/JPAH.2011-0336

212. Wu W, Dasgupta S, Ramirez EE et al (2012) Classification accuracies of physical activities using smartphone motion sensors. J Med Internet Res 14:e130. https://doi.org/10.2196/JMIR.2208

213. Wind DK, Sapiezynski P, Furman MA, Lehmann S (2016) Inferring stop-locations from WiFi. PLoS One 11:e0149105. https://doi.org/10.1371/journal.pone.0149105

214. Geyer K, Ellis DA, Piwek L (2019) A simple location-tracking app for psychological research. Behav Res Methods 51:2840–2846. https://doi.org/10.3758/s13428-018-1164-y

215. Zhou X, Li D (2018) Quantifying multidimensional attributes of human activities at various geographic scales based on smartphone tracking. Int J Health Geogr 17:11. https://doi.org/10.1186/s12942-018-0130-3

216. Ruktanonchai NW, Ruktanonchai CW, Floyd JR, Tatem AJ (2018) Using Google location history data to quantify fine-scale human mobility. Int J Health Geogr 17:28. https://doi.org/10.1186/s12942-018-0150-z

217. Saeb S, Zhang M, Karr CJ et al (2015) Mobile phone sensor correlates of depressive symptom severity in daily life behavior: an exploratory study. J Med Internet Res 17:e175. https://doi.org/10.2196/jmir.4273

218. Clauser SB, Wagner EH, Aiello Bowles EJ et al (2011) Improving modern cancer care through information technology. Am J Prev Med 40:S198–S207. https://doi.org/10.1016/J.AMEPRE.2011.01.014

219. Place S, Blanch-Hartigan D, Rubin C et al (2017) Behavioral indicators on a mobile sensing platform predict clinically validated psychiatric symptoms of mood and anxiety disorders. J Med Internet Res 19:e75. https://doi.org/10.2196/JMIR.6678

220. Peterson SK, Shinn EH, Basen-engquist K et al (2013) Identifying early dehydration risk with home-based sensors during radiation treatment: a feasibility study on patients with head and neck cancer. J Natl Cancer Inst Monogr 2013:162–168. https://doi.org/10.1093/JNCIMONOGRAPHS/LGT016

221. Carter MC, Albar SA, Morris MA et al (2015) Development of a UK online 24-h dietary assessment tool: myfood24. Nutrients 7:4016–4032. https://doi.org/10.3390/nu7064016

222. Liu B, Young H, Crowe FL et al (2011) Development and evaluation of the Oxford WebQ, a low-cost, web-based method for assessment of previous 24 h dietary intakes in large-scale prospective studies. Public Health Nutr 14:1998–2005. https://doi.org/10.1017/S1368980011000942

223. Lo F, Sun Y, Qiu J, Lo B (2018) Food volume estimation based on deep learning view synthesis from a single depth map. Nutrients 10:2005. https://doi.org/10.3390/nu10122005

224. Resende e Silva BV, Rad MG, Cui J et al (2018) A mobile-based diet monitoring system for obesity management. J Health Med Inform 09:307. https://doi.org/10.4172/2157-7420.1000307
225. University of Pittsburgh, Health Sciences Library System Guides (2024) Social & behavioral determinants of health. https://hsls.libguides.com/social-behavioral-determinants-of-health-data. Accessed 27 June 2024
226. Bompelli A, Wang Y, Wan R et al (2021) Social and behavioral determinants of health in the era of artificial intelligence with electronic health records: a scoping review. Health data. Science 2021:9759016. https://doi.org/10.34133/2021/9759016
227. WHO (2024) Social determinants of health. https://www.who.int/health-topics/social-determinants-of-health#tab=tab_1. Accessed 27 June 2024
228. Clark MA, Gurewich D (2017) Integrating measures of social determinants of health into health care encounters: opportunities and challenges. Med Care 55:807–809. https://doi.org/10.1097/MLR.0000000000000788
229. Alley DE, Asomugha CN, Conway PH, Sanghavi DM (2016) Accountable health communities--addressing social needs through medicare and medicaid. N Engl J Med 374:8–11. https://doi.org/10.1056/NEJMP1512532
230. Ash AS, Mick EO, Ellis RP et al (2017) Social determinants of health in managed care payment formulas. JAMA Intern Med 177:1424–1430. https://doi.org/10.1001/JAMAINTERNMED.2017.3317
231. Chen M, Tan X, Padman R (2020) Social determinants of health in electronic health records and their impact on analysis and risk prediction: a systematic review. J Am Med Inform Assoc 27:1764–1773. https://doi.org/10.1093/JAMIA/OCAA143
232. Deferio JJ, Breitinger S, Khullar D et al (2019) Social determinants of health in mental health care and research: a case for greater inclusion. J Am Med Inform Assoc 26:895–899. https://doi.org/10.1093/JAMIA/OCZ049
233. Zhang-James Y, Chen Q, Kuja-Halkola R et al (2020) Machine-learning prediction of comorbid substance use disorders in ADHD youth using Swedish registry data. J Child Psychol Psychiatry 61:1370–1379. https://doi.org/10.1111/JCPP.13226
234. Afshar M, Joyce C, Dligach D et al (2019) Subtypes in patients with opioid misuse: a prognostic enrichment strategy using electronic health record data in hospitalized patients. PLoS One 14:e0219717. https://doi.org/10.1371/journal.pone.0219717
235. Zheng L, Wang O, Hao S et al (2020) Development of an early-warning system for high-risk patients for suicide attempt using deep learning and electronic health records. Transl Psychiatry 10:72. https://doi.org/10.1038/s41398-020-0684-2
236. Chen Q, Zhang-James Y, Barnett EJ et al (2020) Predicting suicide attempt or suicide death following a visit to psychiatric specialty care: a machine learning study using Swedish national registry data. PLoS Med 17:e1003416. https://doi.org/10.1371/journal.pmed.1003416
237. Walsh CG, Ribeiro JD, Franklin JC (2018) Predicting suicide attempts in adolescents with longitudinal clinical data and machine learning. J Child Psychol Psychiatry 59:1261–1270. https://doi.org/10.1111/JCPP.12916
238. Senior M, Burghart M, Yu R et al (2020) Identifying predictors of suicide in severe mental illness: a feasibility study of a clinical prediction rule (Oxford mental illness and suicide tool or OxMIS). Front Psych 11:268. https://doi.org/10.3389/fpsyt.2020.00268
239. Poulymenopoulou M, Papakonstantinou D, Malamateniou F, Vassilacopoulos G (2015) A health analytics semantic ETL service for obesity surveillance. Stud Health Technol Inform 210:840–844
240. Dagliati A, Sacchi L, Tibollo V et al (2018) A dashboard-based system for supporting diabetes care. J Am Med Inform Assoc 25:538–547. https://doi.org/10.1093/JAMIA/OCX159
241. Zhang H, Hosomura N, Shubina M et al (2016) Electronic documentation of lifestyle counselling in primary care is associated with lower risk of cardiovascular events in patients with diabetes. Diabetes 65:A363

242. Davoudi A, Ozrazgat-Baslanti T, Ebadi A et al (2017) Delirium prediction using machine learning models on predictive electronic health records data. In: Proceedings - 2017 IEEE 17th International Conference on Bioinformatics and Bioengineering, BIBE 2017. Washington, DC, USA, pp 568–573

243. Nau C, Ellis H, Huang H et al (2015) Exploring the forest instead of the trees: an innovative method for defining obesogenic and obesoprotective environments. Health Place 35:136–146. https://doi.org/10.1016/J.HEALTHPLACE.2015.08.002

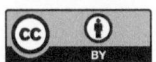

Chapter 2
Electronic Health Data Reuse Purposes

2.1 Electronic Health Data in Public Health

There are many advantages that can arise from the reuse of health data in public health, ranging from the increase in the knowledge base to address health challenges and emergencies to the development of evidence-based medicine to support the decision-making process. As the WHO reminds us in a policy brief: "Data, and the knowledge derived from the use of that data, should be recognized as a global public good, and data-sharing and data reuse should be maximized in ways that are effective, ethical and equitable in order to improve public health" [1]. Public health encompasses a wide variety of different fields (such as environmental health, global health, and social and behavioural health), and in the next section, an overview of electronic health data (EHD) reuse projects that address issues related to epidemiology, surveillance, and occupational health is offered.

2.1.1 Epidemiology

Electronic health data (EHD) present a wide set of opportunities for use in epidemiologic research. Before the 1950s, it was common research practice to use vital statistical data[1] when conducting cross-sectional and time series studies of noninfectious diseases. Drawing causal inference was limited by the lack of longitudinal data until researchers were able to obtain funds to develop cohorts and perform longitudinal follow-ups. However, in the twenty-first century, conducting prospective studies has become time-consuming and costly because of lower research

---

[1] Vital statistics refers to data collected on live births, deaths, migration, foetal deaths, marriages, and divorces. This information is typically obtained through civil registration, an administrative system government's use to record vital events within their populations.

© The Author(s) 2025
F. Cascini, *Secondary Use of Electronic Health Data*, SpringerBriefs in Public Health, https://doi.org/10.1007/978-3-031-88497-9_2

support and participation rates [2]. The increased adoption of electronic health records (EHRs) has been a key factor in the reuse of EHD, as EHRs have begun to generate large volumes of these data, offering a timely alternative to traditional methods of data collection. These databases represent a low-cost source of rich and ample longitudinal data covering large populations that can be used for epidemiologic research. They offer a wide range of applications in epidemiology, since they can also be linked to other types of data and thus yield new insights that would not have been feasible to obtain only by using one source of data. For example, linking EHR data with genomic or biobank data allows researchers to study the genetic basis of diseases and responses to treatments [3]. Linking them with registries of certain diseases (such as trauma registries) can improve both data accuracy and completeness and provide an excellent source of longitudinal data, which can be particularly beneficial for chronic disease management, such as diabetes or cancer, where long-term outcomes are critical [4].

The reuse of health data in epidemiology can be appreciated in several contexts, from those related to communicable diseases to those related to risk stratification and prevention. The most common use cases are based on the reuse of EHR (however, other types of EHD can be reused), and these examples are presented in the following paragraphs.

2.1.1.1   Genomic Epidemiology

Genomics plays a crucial role in both pathogen diagnosis and epidemiology. Pathogen sequencing has been utilized for decades to track viral outbreaks, starting from studies on hantavirus in the United States [5] and human immunodeficiency virus (HIV) in the UK [6]. In recent years, this methodology has been expanded to include bacterial pathogens and is now referred to as genomic epidemiology, a field that covers everything from population dynamics to tracing individual transmission events during outbreaks [7]. Most transmission-focused studies have been retrospective, with only a small proportion being conducted in real time as cases are diagnosed. For example, one study conducted a real-time assessment of whole-genome sequencing (WGS) for the routine typing and monitoring of verocytotoxin-producing *Escherichia coli* (VTEC). In Denmark, the Statens Serum Institut (SSI) regularly receives all suspected VTEC isolates. As part of Denmark's routine surveillance, hospitals sent suspected VTEC isolates from infected patients to SSI for confirmation and further phenotypic and molecular analyses. All incoming isolates were concurrently subjected to WGS, after which real-time bioinformatics analysis and real-time clustering of the isolates were performed, which was in agreement with the epidemiological findings, and were thus able to discriminate between sporadic and outbreak isolates [8]. Other data highlight the potential of this technology for real-time investigations of bacterial outbreaks. Another study utilized conventional molecular techniques alongside WGS to examine an outbreak of *Legionella pneumophila* in a major Australian hospital. Typing these isolates through sequence-based methods and virulence gene profiling did not successfully distinguish between outbreak and nonoutbreak isolates. WGS was conducted on isolates collected during the outbreak as well as on unrelated isolates from the Public Health Microbiology reference collection and managed to distinguish outbreak isolates from those that were neither temporally nor spatially related to the outbreak [9]. The reuse of genomic data has also proven to be valuable in supporting food-borne outbreaks. WGS managed to assess a *Salmonella enteritidis* phage type 14b (PT14b) outbreak in the UK, which occurred at the same time as outbreaks in other European Union Member States. Food traceback investigations in the UK and other affected European countries revealed a link between the outbreaks and chicken eggs from a German company. WGS conducted on isolates from UK and European cases, as well as from implicated UK premises and German eggs, revealed a high degree of similarity among the isolates. Together with the food traceback data, these results confirmed that the UK outbreak was linked with the German producer [10].

Another example of the use of genomic data for the purposes of epidemiology and surveillance is the initiative known as One Health, which was launched in 2004. One Health provider aspires to provide effective approaches to disease surveillance, management, and prevention while recognizing the connections between human health, domestic animal health, and wildlife health and disease [11]. In this course of action, the One Health Initiative seeks to address the need for an integrated system that includes environmental, animal, and human monitoring as crucial areas of surveillance for protecting human health, a goal in which genomics plays an important part. While the objective of using integrated surveillance data to predict outbreaks remains years away, One Health studies are already employing genomic epidemiology tools and techniques to investigate ongoing outbreaks. The integration of genomic data with information from advanced One Health surveillance systems may support the identification of population expansions or cross-species transmissions that could trigger the onset of a human health event. For example, the genome sequences of a raccoon-associated rabies virus (RRV) variant, combined with detailed geographic information and data from Canadian and US wildlife rabies vaccination programmes, revealed that multiple cross-border invasions were responsible for the spread of RRV into Canada, causing outbreaks in several provinces [12]. This discovery prompted renewed public health efforts to combat rabies [13]. Another early study that integrated detailed wildlife and livestock movement data with phylodynamic analysis of a bacterial pathogen revealed that cross-species transmission from an elk reservoir was the source of increasing *Brucella abortus* infections in nearby livestock [14]. As brucellosis is the most common zoonotic disease in humans, control programmes for this infection could greatly benefit from such a One Health approach [15]. All these efforts to integrate health and genomic epidemiology provide a basis of work that could derive useful epidemiological insights, including signals of population expansion, proof of transmission within and between animal reservoirs and humans, and epidemiological analysis of a pathogen's early expansion [16].

2.1.1.2 Assembling Research Cohorts

EHR data can be used in epidemiological research to select cohorts and specific groups of patients. For example, Kaiser Permanente in the United States established several EHR-based cohorts [17–20]. One of them was a nested case–control study within a cohort of infants (407 cases with at least one autism spectrum disorder [ASD] diagnosis and 2095 controls), which concluded that maternal autoimmune disorders occurring around the time of pregnancy are unlikely to play a significant role in the risk of autism [17]. Another large case–control study nested within a cohort of singleton term infants (338 patients diagnosed with ASD and 1817 controls) reported that neonatal hyperbilirubinemia is not a risk factor for ASD [17]. Another example was the Chronic Hepatitis Cohort Study (CHeCS), a dynamic, prospective, longitudinal, observational cohort study established to evaluate the clinical impact of chronic viral hepatitis in the United States. This study analysed EHRs from over 1.6 million adult patients seen between January 2006 and December 2010 at 4 integrated US healthcare systems and identified 2202 patients with chronic hepatitis B virus (HBV) infection. Baseline data on demographics, hospitalizations, and mortality from CHeCS underscore the significant health burden of chronic viral hepatitis in the United States, particularly among individuals born between 1945 and 1964 [21]. The use of EHRs also provides an opportunity to design a large-scale prospective study (known as the Diabetes Study of Northern California [DISTANCE]), which included 20,000 diabetic patients and has investigated a wide range of issues such as diabetes outcomes among Asians and Pacific Islanders [22] and the influence of neighbourhood deprivation on cardiometabolic health [23]. There are also examples of collaboration between researchers from multiple health systems; some examples include the HMO Research Network, which started this type of research in 1994 [24], and the Consortium on Safe Labor [25–28], which performs research on delivery and birth data from EHRs from 19 hospitals and studies the effects of different factors (such as acute air pollution exposure to normo/hypertensive women and preeclampsia) on pregnancy and neonatal outcomes.

2.1.1.3 Validation of the Results of Smaller Studies

Big EHR data are used to validate the results of smaller studies. This is particularly useful in cases where smaller studies have reported inconsistent results, such as in the case of the association between midlife body mass index (BMI) and later-life dementia. Qizilbash et al. [29] conducted a retrospective cohort study involving a cohort of 1,958,191 individuals from the UK Clinical Practice Research Datalink (CPRD), consisting of people aged 40 years and older with recorded BMIs between 1992 and 2007. After employing Poisson regression to calculate dementia incidence rates for each BMI category, they showed that being underweight in middle and old age is associated with an increased risk of dementia over a two-decade period. These results challenge the hypothesis that middle-aged obesity increases the risk of developing dementia later in life [29]. Another study compared the short-term respiratory morbidity associated with late preterm births (34–36 weeks gestation) with that associated with term births in the United States. This retrospective study included data from 12 institutions and 19 hospitals, encompassing 233,844 deliveries between 2002 and 2008. The key outcomes were neonates admitted to neonatal intensive care units (NICUs) due to respiratory issues. Multivariate logistic regression adjusted for factors influencing respiratory outcomes indicated that late preterm births had a significantly greater risk of respiratory distress syndrome and other respiratory complications than did term deliveries. This evidence highlights the vulnerability of late preterm infants and underscores the importance of monitoring and potentially intervening to reduce the risk of respiratory complications in this population [25]. Similarly, conclusions have been drawn from small-scale studies from fertility clinics regarding the association between celiac disease and infertility. This finding was not supported by a large population-based study of women in the UK, which used data from The Health Improvement Network (THIN) database. A cohort of 2,426,225 women, recorded between 1990 and 2013, was analysed for age-specific rates of newly recorded fertility problems, comparing women with and without a celiac disease (CD) diagnosis. The researchers stratified the data on the basis of whether CD was diagnosed before or after the onset of fertility issues and controlled for factors such as sociodemographics, comorbidities, and time periods. The key finding of the study was that women with CD did not exhibit a greater overall likelihood of infertility than women without CD did. However, women aged 25–39 years who had been diagnosed with CD had a slightly higher rate of reported fertility problems. This suggests that while CD might not universally increase the risk of infertility, there may be a notable association in specific age groups or under certain conditions [30].

2.1.1.4   Environmental and Social Epidemiology

Environmental and social epidemiologists can use EHR data to study patients distributed across a wide range of physical, built, and social environments. Since patient addresses are checked and updated at the regular level, researchers can use location-specific data to investigate proximity to hazards and their health implications. For example, EHR studies have investigated the physical environment (e.g. air pollution, green space) and its health effects (e.g. hypertension, diabetes, migraines) [26, 28, 31–33]. For example, a study conducted by a research group from the Netherlands explored the link between physician-assessed morbidity and green space in residential areas. Morbidity data were obtained from the electronic medical records of 195 general practitioners (GPs) across 96 Dutch practices, covering 345,143 individuals. Green space percentages within 1 km and 3 km radii around postal code coordinates were calculated via an existing database. Multilevel logistic regression was used, adjusting for demographic and socioeconomic factors. The results revealed that 15 of 24 disease clusters had a lower prevalence in areas with more green space within 1 km, with the strongest associations for anxiety and depression, especially among children and those with lower socioeconomic status in

slightly urban areas [34]. There are also studies that have explored the health implications of the built environment, such as land use (street connectivity, population
density), food (density of fast-food restaurants, food deserts), and physical activity
environments (e.g. access parks, diversity of physical activity establishments) [33,
35–41]. For example, studies have demonstrated the utility of using EHR data for
conducting large-scale population-based epidemiologic research [40] and that
incorporating community data into EHRs enhances the potential for secondary use
of EHR data to study and address obesity prevention and other major public health
concerns [39]. Moreover, the regression analyses of these cross-sectional studies,
which are based on EHR data, uniformly point to the importance of the built environment and children's weight status [33, 37, 39, 40] and that built environment
characteristics that may increase walkability are associated with lower BMI [37].
Finally, other research groups reported that other environmental exposures affect
human health by analysing EHR data. One study reported that exposure to unconventional natural gas development activity increased the chance of preterm birth.
This was a retrospective cohort study using electronic health record data from 9384
mothers linked to 10,946 neonates in the Geisinger Health System between January
2009 and January 2013. The cumulative exposure to unconventional natural gas
development was estimated via an inverse-distance squared model, which accounts
for the distance to the mother's home, as well as the dates, durations of well pad
development, drilling, hydraulic fracturing, and production volume during pregnancy. Another study evaluated the health-related impact of another important environmental factor—the distance from coal-abandoned mine lands—represented by
ten contextual metrics at the community level. Cross-sectional and longitudinal
multilevel analyses of data obtained from 28,000 diabetic primary care patients at
the Geisinger Clinic revealed an association between abandoned coal mine lands
and higher levels of HbA1c [38].

2.1.1.5 Research on Stigmatized Conditions

Stigmatized conditions are health issues or personal characteristics that are viewed
negatively or socially disapproved of by society. People with these conditions often
face prejudice, discrimination, and judgement, which can lead to feelings of shame,
isolation, and a reluctance to seek treatment or disclose their condition [42]. This is
why research on stigmatized conditions may face challenges due to difficulties in
patient recruitment and follow-up. Some examples of such conditions include mental disorders, AIDS, venereal diseases, leprosy, and certain skin diseases. This is
why reusing EHD (in particular, EHRs) has many advantages, especially because it
addresses the problem of patient recruitment. For example, one Rwanda study analysed EHR data and information from community health workers to compare the
mental health of HIV-positive children, children living with HIV-positive parents,
and HIV-unaffected children. The use of these data enabled this research group to
conclude that children living with HIV-positive parents need the same mental health
services as infected children themselves do [43]. There are also efforts to utilize

EHRs and EMRs to identify people experiencing homelessness with greater precision to support interventions at both the patient and population levels aimed at addressing health inequities [44, 45]. For example, one study developed an enhanced EHR registry to improve the identification of persons experiencing homelessness within a safety net healthcare system. The study compared patients identified as experiencing homelessness in 2021, stratifying them by the method of identification (i.e. through registration data sources versus the new EHR registry criteria). The results showed that commonly used methods for identifying persons experiencing homelessness in healthcare systems may underestimate the population and introduce reporting biases, thus highlighting the need to recognize alternative identification methods to more comprehensively and inclusively identify persons experiencing homelessness for targeted interventions [46].

2.1.2 Surveillance

Public health surveillance started in the late 1800s with the spread of infectious diseases at the time. As a key action of public health practice, it is based on collections of information driving interventions to address population diseases in general, from communicable diseases to chronic diseases, sexually transmitted diseases, vaccine-preventable diseases and others [47].

With the spread of mobile phone usage worldwide, this change has contributed dramatically to increasing the amount of available data from multiple sources (social media, health apps, etc.), including data relevant from a public health and medical perspective. Although, as signalled by Van Panhuis et al., barriers still exist in terms of the technical, motivational, economic, ethical, legal, and political aspects, this does not undermine the potential of EHD for public health; moreover, it justifies the need to accelerate a process that has continued behind the rapid pace of technological advances today [48].

The increased use of EHRs in the United States provides new opportunities for the future of public health surveillance. In fact, experiences such as the Electronic Medical Record Support for Public Health (ESPnet) surveillance platform have been able to generate modules for a wide range of diseases, from tuberculosis to type 2 diabetes. Although some challenges have been identified, especially in the case of requiring new installations and updated detection algorithms to properly function to accommodate changes in treatments, these challenges could be overcome or reduced in the future with the implementation of standardization practices by the Centers for Disease Control and Prevention (CDC) or other organizations [47].

In a world where post-market medical device surveillance is still a challenge faced by regulatory agencies, healthcare providers, and manufacturers, EHD surveillance may offer an opportunity to follow up device indicators at a greater scale and lower cost than traditional methods do. This potential is increased by the merging and interaction of new technologies that leverage the potential of EHD for multiple surveillance purposes, including the scaling up of local data for regional or national surveillance purposes and the filling of large or outdated data gaps with the use of EHD for analysis purposes. Among the technologies that leverage EHD for surveillance, natural language processing (NLP), machine learning (ML), and other algorithms, such as the naive Bayes algorithm, are examples of different technologies that are surging and being developed and validated because of data usage for surveillance. Moreover, with the rapid surge of technology and increasing quality of data every day, more technologies will likely become part of the future of EHD for surveillance.

In fact, the use of modern ML technologies may support the use and analysis of increasingly complex information derived from text and other sources, thus increasing the potential use of EHD for surveillance and other purposes [49]. Some other AI tools, such as existing modern deep learning techniques that are in the research phase, have been able to recognize patient outcomes from clinical notes without the need for manually labelled training data. These state-of-the-art learning methods have already been developed and validated, showing a precision of up to 96% for hip replacement records. The information gathered was able to detect important indicators such as variation in outcomes between implants, higher or lower rates of hip mentions, and others [49].

Finally, EHD may present an opportunity for research in areas where there is a knowledge gap or when only outdated information is available due to a lack of active surveillance. In the case of dementia in Spain, outdated information from 2010 led researchers to address the validity of EHD recorded during primary care for research purposes. Using information from the System for the Development of Research in Primary Care (SIDAIP), which contains anonymized information from >80% of the population in Catalonia, researchers investigated whether the dementia diagnoses made by general practitioners (GPs) during primary care were valid enough to be used for research purposes.

After contrasting the results from GPs with those of specialists via survey, they were able to estimate the incidence and prevalence of dementia in the population with a positive predictive value (PPV) of 91%, similar to face-to-face studies conducted in Spain and confirming the potential of using EHDs obtained during primary care consultations for dementia research [50]. This could therefore provide an opportunity to investigate even further the potential of primary care data to shape research as well as policy actions not only for dementia but also for diseases or conditions for which data gaps exist but for which primary care EHD is available and could provide insights at a lower cost and higher scale.

- **FDA Sentinel System**

  Since its inception in 2009, the Sentinel System has played a crucial role in the FDA's capability for surveillance. EHD is used to increase the ability of post-market surveillance for many purposes, including evaluating the safety of post-market products. The Medicare Fee for Service (FFS) data, as well as those of partners from national and local health plans, are among the data contributors for Sentinel. Other partners include PCORnet, EHR-based organizations, and networks. During the COVID-19 outbreak in the country and to address the FDA's anticipated data and analytical needs early in the outbreak response, Sentinel developed a comprehensive approach that incorporated early aggregated data sources, a quickly updated database, and a validated algorithm to identify patients with COVID-19 in administrative claims data [51].

- **EHD analysis is a cost-effective solution, PHINEX case study.**
  EHD analysis provides more cost-effective approaches as technological advances and data analysis frameworks evolve each day. For local surveillance systems, this could mean having an effective approach for tackling emerging public health concerns both at local and regional scales at a reduced cost and with opportunities for early interceptions when needed, as may be the case for childhood obesity. As an example of its potential, research using data extracted from the Public Health Information Exchange (PHINEX) database, which contains information from children and adolescents (2–19 years), was transformed from deidentified EHRs into a two-step procedure that was able to adjust for missing data and weights for a national population distribution, thus resulting in estimates comparable to those of the National Health and Nutrition Examination Survey (NHANES), which were produced with the need for considerably more resources. This highlights the opportunity for EHRs to use data to address regional disparities and support early intervention at a lower cost and higher speed [52].

- **Communicable Disease Surveillance**
  Algorithms could serve as excellent tools to detect cases of communicable diseases and inform appropriate preventive actions in the case of epidemics. Initiatives on this topic have been carried out for diseases such as tuberculosis, acute viral hepatitis, and sexually transmitted diseases, achieving considerably high sensitivity and positive predictive values (PPVs) in some cases [47].

- **Surveillance of Chronic Diseases**
  There are fewer current cases of EHD use for chronic diseases than for communicable diseases. Examples of this use include the development of a clinical algorithm for diabetes types I and II developed within the ESPnet using ICD-9 codes, which are derived from prescriptions of oral hypoglycaemic agents or insulin. The algorithm had a sensitivity of 97% and a PPV of 88%. Fundamentally, EHD for chronic disease surveillance is different from the fact that it does not require traceability for individual cases; therefore, the information collected does not need to be identifiable [47].

- **Post-market Surveillance**
  To bridge the gap between the concept and the practical reality of employing electronic health data for post-market surveillance, three groundbreaking research projects have been proposed at the moment: (1) the Observational Medical Outcomes Partnership (OMOP), established in the United States by the FDA, the National Institutes of Health, and the drug industry lobbying group Pharmaceutical Research and Manufacturers of America (Pharmacoepidemiological Research on Therapeutic Outcomes by a European Consortium) held by the European Medicines Agency (EMA), and (3) the Sentinel Initiative, a national medical product safety surveillance system intro-

duced by the FDA in 2009. At this point in time, all three initiatives have finished their initial cycles, with the OMOP initiative being the most extensive and systematic of those, with more than 50 M participants from the US population, including Medicaid, Medicare, and employ-based insured families.

In addition to these efforts, there is still no credible evidence on the capacity of EHD to provide robust and reliable active surveillance, nevertheless, as the growth potential is substantial, as well as the cost effectiveness of the procedure in comparison with, for example, clinical trials cost millions of dollars, the use of financial and other resources to be allocated for addressing current issues of reliability, reproducibility, and statistical standards, among others, remains a priority to capitalize on this potential in the future [53].

- **Genomic Pathogen Surveillance**
  Global Pneumococcal Sequencing (GPS) Project. The Global Pneumococcal Sequencing (GPS) project was initiated in 2011 with the primary goal of creating a global picture of pneumococcal evolution during vaccine introductions in low-income and middle-income countries via whole-genome sequencing. By the end of 2019, the project had sequenced >26,000 pneumococcal isolates from >50 countries.

  Barriers encountered in the process include the lack of microbiological expertise, as well as motivations and limitations from partners in the project, with some partners being content with the contribution of culture samples to the project, while other partners taking a more desirable and actively involved attitude referred to developing local genomics capacity and a desire to generate local data in a way that could be integrated with the global database. Although the second attitude should be encouraged, it is important to note that flexibility is key to not lead to partner disengagement and therefore a weakening of the surveillance data captured.

  Among the needs highlighted by the outputs of the GPS project over almost a decade, several could be translated into multiple disease fields: (1) Increased need for geographical coverage, especially in countries with a high disease burden. (2) Increased support for local data generation and analysis provided by capacity building and bioinformatics training. (3) Increased engagement with policy makers to communicate the value of data and study findings for decision-making, in this case, for pneumococcal disease prevention. In 2020, the GPS project started its transition into the GPS2 project [54, 55].

- **PulseNet, an example of a national pilot program with international scalability.**
  PulseNet USA was established in 1996 as the national molecular surveillance network for foodborne infections. The network's goal was to use pulse field gel electrophoresis (PFGE) and a nationwide database of PFGE patterns to quickly identify epidemics caused by foodborne viruses. In 1002, the 50 states reached their goal of complete national participation. By 2005, the network included 8 food safety regulatory laboratories, 4 nations, 3 cities, and 65 cooperating public health laboratories. To identify outbreaks, it connects and incorporates cases of food-borne, water-borne, and other illnesses [56]. Owing to PulseNet's success

and scaling potential, PulseNet International is currently present in a variety of locations, including the United States, Canada, Europe, Asia Pacific, the Middle East, Latin America, and the Caribbean.

Whole-genome sequencing (WGS) for food-borne sequencing is currently being implemented by PulseNet International in all public health laboratories worldwide. This is because WGS, which offers the following benefits, will improve the global response to outbreaks and diseases caused by food-borne pathogens. It can be standardized, has good epidemiologic concordance, generates data that are portable and simple to compare, does not necessitate formal bioinformatics expertise, and permits the creation of analysis tools that are available to the public. For this purpose and to make it easier for members to share and compare data, PulseNet International is creating, certifying, and distributing standard analytic processes. It is also building quality control systems and standardized terminology [57–59].

2.1.3   Occupational Health

In occupational health, workplace injury and illness data from physician reporting, employer records and workers compensation claims have been long-standing resources for research and surveillance. In Europe, countries such as Scandinavia have a long tradition of linking cohort studies to register data to gain insight into predictors of sick leave and work disability. A key aim of exploiting these data is to improve the capacity to predict and prevent injury and disease in the workplace [60]. Moreover, with the surge of new occupational risks and hazards emerging because of societal change and new technology implementation, a change from the occupational health approach used for industrial medicine to the digitization of work becomes necessary [61]. Some examples of reuse include the following:

- **Total Worker Health:** The concept of "total worker health", introduced in 2011 by the US federal agency named National Institute for Occupational Safety and Health (NIOSH), has brought a new dimension of care to occupational health, therefore not focusing on the prevention of injury and illness in the workplace but rather moving one step forward into the well-being of workers. This change in vision of the application of occupational health also provides new opportunities for occupational health workers to have a greater impact on the health of populations.
- **Infodemiology and infoveillance:** The use of big data in occupational health provides new opportunities for the application of technologies to support and promote the health of working populations. Given the rapid surge in availability of data, terms related to its use as "infodemiology", defined as the combination of information and epidemiology, and "infoveillance", information + surveillance, are the result of an understanding of the importance that data, including big data, will have in the future of health for populations, including those in the

workplace, and how this information could shape health by influencing factors such as the social determinants of health of workers.

- **Contribution to public health:** If institutions such as occupational health services (OHS) and others properly capitalize on the increase in data available, data could serve to promote well-designed occupational health strategies that, if developed at a national or even international level, could significantly contribute to public health goals. This has a significant influence in a society where a sizeable portion of the population spends not only a reasonable number of hours each day but also a significant portion of their lifetime. Therefore, it can also be concluded that occupational health has a significant effect on public health objectives, and data could be used to influence future generations' health.

2.2   Electronic Health Data for Institutional Activities and Policy Making

Several initiatives based on EHD reuse have been established over the years by eminent global institutions such as the World Health Organization (WHO), continental institutions such as the European Centre for Disease Prevention and Control (ECDC), and some regional institutions such as the National Institute for Health and Care Excellence (NICE) in the UK. Regardless of the type of institution—regardless of whether it operates on a global, continental, or regional level—it has the same goal: to propose policies and activities that will enable better health-related outcomes at the population level. Through many initiatives, they focus on EHD reuse. Some of the aims are strengthening defences against infectious diseases by conducting surveillance, risk assessment, and epidemic intelligence; working on the capacity to respond to health threats or prevent disease outbreaks; and setting health standards and health policies that aim to improve healthcare systems.

2.2.1   The European Centre for Disease Prevention and Control (ECDC) Initiatives

The European Centre for Disease Prevention and Control (ECDC) is an EU agency established in 2005, with a mission to strengthen Europe's defences against infectious diseases by identifying, assessing, and communicating about potential threats to human health. The ECDC established partnerships with European national health protection bodies to develop disease surveillance and early warning systems at the continental level. To achieve the final goal, the ECDC collaborates with experts throughout Europe to develop and publish scientific opinions regarding the risks associated with current/emerging infectious diseases. Specifically, some of the tasks associated with this field of mission include searching, collating, evaluating, and disseminating scientific/technical data; providing scientific opinions and scientific and technical assistance; and informing the Commission, Member States, Community agencies, and public health-oriented international organizations in a timely manner. There are several initiatives of the ECDC relying on EHD reuse that play a crucial role in public health by enhancing disease surveillance, enabling rapid detection and monitoring of public health threats, promoting vaccination to prevent vaccine-preventable diseases, and addressing key challenges such as antimicrobial resistance (AMR).

- **EpiPulse - the European surveillance portal for infectious diseases**
  EpiPulse [62] is an online portal launched in June 2021 that integrates several previously independent surveillance systems (the European Surveillance System [TESSy], the five Epidemic Intelligence Information System [EPIS] platforms, and the Threat Tracking Tool [TTT]). This online portal is used by European public health authorities and partner organizations for collecting, analysing, sharing, and discussing infectious disease data to detect threats, perform monitoring, risk assessment, and prepare for an outbreak response.
  This portal functions such that experts from the EU/EEA and non-EU countries within the ECDC's cooperation framework, ECDC staff, and representatives of European authorities, and international organizations can report and analyse cases of infectious diseases and pathogens that may represent public health threats in the EU/EEA. It facilitates interdisciplinary collaboration by connecting experts from different sectors via a One Health approach.
- **ECDC Vaccine Scale**
  The Vaccine Scheduler is an interactive tool that presents vaccination schedules for individual EU/EEA countries and specific age groups and thus enables comparisons depending on the country or disease (for all or selected countries). However, it is also suggested that the national competent bodies consult for the most up-to-date schedules, even though this platform has been continuously monitored.
  Some of the applications of this tool included the analysis of recommended and mandatory vaccination schedules from over 30 European countries due to the major 2016 measles epidemic that affected EU/EEA countries. The study obtained information on current national immunization programmes from the "Vaccine Scheduler" to derive informed decisions regarding the trending measles public health threat [63]. In addition to this case, it was also applied in the case of Human Papilloma Virus vaccination schedules [64] and for analysing vaccination policies for migrants in 32 EU/EEA countries and Switzerland [65].
- **Antimicrobial consumption dashboard (ESAC-Net)**
  ESAC-Net represents the EU/EEA reference data obtained from the European Surveillance of Antimicrobial Consumption Network (ESAC-Net) and is reported through the TESSy surveillance system [66]. This interactive dashboard contains data and trends for the EU/EEA and individual countries for both the community and hospital sectors. It also includes antimicrobial surveillance tools that enable the visualization of different quality indicators relevant for antibiotic

consumption. This dashboard, for example, enables analyses that can inform policy making regarding antibiotic prescriptions and address the issue of antimicrobial resistance (both at the network level and at the country level) either by focusing on general groups of antibiotics [67] or on specific types, such as quinolones [68].

- **The European Surveillance System (TESSy)**
  TESSy is an ECDC surveillance system that facilitates the collection, analysis, and dissemination of European surveillance data on infectious diseases [69]. The EU Member States are obligated to provide the ECDC with relevant available scientific and technical data in a timely manner. The data holder and controller is the ECDC, which also performs technical implementations related to data publication and the granting of data access in accordance with this policy. After validation, the data are published in the Surveillance Atlas of Infectious Diseases on the ECDC website [70]. The difference between the Surveillance Atlas and TESSy is in the type of analyses and presentations they provide. While a good epidemiological overview of infectious diseases in the EU/EEA can be provided by the atlas, the analyses can only be given by year. On the other hand, TESSy data can be used for performing analyses for shorter time periods, which makes them more informative.

  The existence of such a database and collaboration enables the performance of epidemiological analyses of serious infectious threats, such as invasive meningococcal disease (IMD). One study described the epidemiology of IMD in EU/EEA countries covering the period between 2004 and 2014 to explore trends depending on serogroup and age and to compare country trends based on the introduction of the meningococcal C conjugate (MCC) vaccine [71]. These findings confirmed that routine MCC vaccination decreased the infection rates caused by serogroup C. The study also reported that vaccination against serogroup B in the first year of life could reduce the burden of IMD caused by this serogroup. This is only one example of a serogroup-specific change trend that emphasizes the need for high-quality surveillance data to perform accurate assessments of changing epidemiology (in this case, IMD) to measure the effectiveness and impact of implemented vaccine programmes and inform accurate policy making. Some other examples include investigations of Campylobacter seasonality across Europe for a defined period by using this system [72] or providing information about influenza seasonal surveillance [73], among many other examples.

2.2.2 European Medicines Agency (EMA) Initiatives

The European Medicines Agency (EMA) is aimed at fostering scientific excellence in the process of evaluating and supervising medicines in the EU (both for animal and human health). One of its tasks is to enable timely access of patients to new medicines and to support the development of medicines that will benefit them. The agency implements a variety of regulatory mechanisms such as providing support for early access, providing scientific advice, assisting in the development of protocols, and providing quality/safety/efficacy guidelines for medical tests, among others. It also supports research and innovation among pharmaceutical micro, small-, and medium-sized enterprises. The agency's evaluations of marketing authorization applications submitted through the centralized procedure provide the basis for the authorization of medicines in Europe [74]. There are several EMA projects that rely on EHD reuse. In particular, initiatives guided by the EMA aim to increase medicine safety and reduce harmful drug-related events by monitoring real-world data (EHD) at the population level. They are also focused on ensuring adequate response and preparedness in times of health-related crisis and thereby act to ensure better overall health outcomes for populations. These initiatives are presented in the following paragraphs.

2.2.2.1 Pharmacovigilance (EudraVigilance)

This system allows adverse reaction information management and analysis for the medicines that received authorization or for which clinical testing has been performed in the EEA [75]. EudraVigilance started operation in December 2001, and the government's access to the database was performed by the EudraVigilance Access Policy. The EMA operates the system in front of the EU medicine regulatory network. The role of EudraVigilance is to provide electronic information exchange on medicine safety between EMAs and different authorities (national competent authorities, marketing authorization holders, and clinical trial sponsors in the EEA). This facilitates early detection/evaluation of potential safety signals and better information about products authorized in the EEA. More specifically, this system includes a safety and message-processing mechanism that is fully automated (using XML-based messaging) and a large pharmacovigilance database that has query and tracking functions. It complies with the formats and standards of the International Council on Harmonization of Technical Requirements for Registration of Pharmaceuticals for Human Use (ICH). After the full implementation of pharmacovigilance legislation in 2010, further enhancements were implemented to EudraVigilance, and a major revision was performed of its access policy, considering the use of the new individual case safety report standard developed by the ICH and the International Organization for Standardization [75, 76].

Some of the latest examples of utilization of this system were for assessing, monitoring, and comparing the adverse reactions caused by COVID-19 vaccines across Europe, namely the occurrence of cerebral vein thrombosis associated with thrombocytopenia after the first dose of the adenoviral vector vaccines CHADOX1 NCOV-19 and AD26. COV2 [77]. Similarly, another study performed a retrospective descriptive analysis of the adverse events reported after receiving the Moderna, Pfizer, and Oxford-AstraZeneca COVID-19 vaccines, which were submitted to the EudraVigilance database. The focus was again on thrombotic events [78]. The EudraVigilance database was utilized to assess other vaccine-related adverse events, such as the occurrence of autoimmune disorders after receiving adjuvanted (Celtura™, Fluval P™, Focetria™, and Pandemrix™) and nonadjuvanted (Cantgrip™, Celvapan™, and Panenza™) pandemic influenza A/H1N1 vaccines. The aim was to determine whether adjuvant vaccines were associated with a higher rate of adverse events [79]. This database allows monitoring of post-marketing surveillance but also investigates the consistency of the disproportionality signals reported in the EudraVigilance database and another database (in this case, the American Food and Drug Administration Adverse Event Reporting System) [80]. This database can also be used for assessing the rates of medication abuse, misuse, and dependency, such as in the case of opioids [81]. This study used data from two pharmacovigilance datasets (EudraVigilance and the FDA Adverse Events Reporting System) to identify and describe these issues. A descriptive analysis of the selected adverse drug reactions was performed, and pharmacovigilance signal measures (i.e. reporting odds ratios, proportional reporting ratios) were computed for preferred terms of abuse, misuse, dependence, and withdrawal, as well as preferred terms eventually related to them (e.g. aggression) [81].

2.2.3 European Health Emergency Preparedness and Response (HERA) Initiatives

The Health Emergency Preparedness and Response (HERA) department operates to prevent, detect, and rapidly respond to health emergencies. It was created in the aftermath of the COVID-19 pandemic to predict possible threats and health crises by gathering intelligence and developing capacities for response. In the case of an emergency, HERA is responsible for ensuring the development, production, and distribution of medical countermeasures, which were found to be lacking during the initial phase of the response to the COVID-19 pandemic. HERA began operating as a new European Commission Directorate-General in September 2021, and it oversees the Commission's policies related to public health. It is envisioned to be the key pillar in the European Health Union's emergency response and preparedness.

In October 2022, the European Health Union was concluded, after which several regulations were adopted: the Regulation on serious cross-border threats to health, the Regulation on the Extended Mandate of the European Centre for Disease Prevention and Control (ECDC), and the Council Regulation on the Emergency Framework regarding Medical Countermeasures (the Emergency Framework Regulation). The adoption of these Regulations granted extra powers to HERA [82]. With respect to HERA's activities relying on electronic health data reuse, HERA's mandate for the period between 2022 and 2027 should address cross-border health threats and provide associated medical countermeasures such as crisis-related vaccines, medicines, personal protective equipment, diagnostics, active pharmaceutical ingredients, and critical raw materials. After consulting with the EMA and ECDC, HERA identified three threat categories that were recognized as top priorities: (i) pathogens with high pandemic potential; (ii) chemical, biological, radiological, and nuclear (CBRN) threats originating from accidental or deliberate release; and (iii) antimicrobial resistance (AMR) [83].

Furthermore, the HERA IT platform is under development. This digital system will enable the gathering of intelligence by utilizing a wide range of data that will aid decision-making processes related to medical countermeasures, namely forecasting, developing, and testing particular possible scenarios. This platform provides outputs generated from ECDC-operated epidemiological surveillance networks and epidemic intelligence systems and from medicine-related forecasts and information gathered by the EMA.

In fact, EMAs, ECDCs, and HERAs collaborate tightly to provide an efficient response to crisis situations (across Europe and around the world) during their mandate. While HERA has a central role in identifying, developing, procuring, stockpiling, and deploying medical countermeasures during health emergencies, ECDC and EMA provide the intelligence that is required for carrying out all these tasks. For example, HERA relies on ECDC outputs (especially from epidemiological surveillance networks and their risk assessments on communicable disease and threats), which are then combined with either their own collected data or surveillance data from other sources and thus rapidly respond to health threats that need medical countermeasures.

For example, in May 2022, the ECDC epidemic intelligence detected signals of a monkeypox outbreak, HERA (after receiving advice from the EMA), which located the available authorized and unauthorized monkeypox treatments and vaccines. Afterwards, aligned with its mandate, HERA collected information from national competent authorities and the industry related to therapeutic and vaccine supply and demand (after consulting the HERA Board). This allowed HERA to respond rapidly and efficiently to the ongoing crisis by purchasing and distributing vaccines to EU/EEA countries and by organizing joint acquisitions for antiviral purchases.

2.2.4   The US Centers for Disease Control and Prevention (CDC) Initiatives

The Centers for Disease Control and Prevention (CDC) is one of the leading organizations that aims to protect public health by deriving science- and evidence-based decisions [84]. It has a role in ensuring America's health, safety, and security and in fighting diseases that either occur at home/abroad, are chronic or acute, and are for curing or preventing. To achieve this goal, the CDC collects and provides critical scientific information that can enable both protection against health threats and response when such threats occur. The CDC's projects, which rely on electronic health data reuse, include the following.

- **The BEAM (Bacteria, Enterics, Amoeba, and Mycotics) Dashboard [85]**

This is an online interactive tool that provides access and visualization of data retrieved from the System for Enteric Disease Response, Investigation, and Coordination (SEDRIC). This dashboard can be used to explore the trends of pathogens together with serotype details that can help in curbing illness-related burdens (both due to food and animal contact). Currently, the focus of the dashboard is on data for *Salmonella*, Shiga toxin-producing *E. coli* (STEC), *Shigella* and *Campylobacter* bacteria; antimicrobial resistance; and multistate outbreaks, and additional pathogen- and epidemiology-related data will be included in the future. Examples of visualizations can be found at this address [85]. The datasets are public (without any restrictions) and can be downloaded upon request (while previews and visualizations are immediately accessible).

- **The Disability and Health Data System (DHDS)**
  The prevalence of disability status and types relies on data obtained from the Disability and Health Data System (DHDS). This online source provides state-level data from adults diagnosed with some of the six functional disability types: cognitive (serious difficulty concentrating, remembering, or making decisions), hearing (serious difficulty hearing or deaf), mobility (serious difficulty walking or climbing stairs), vision (serious difficulty seeing), self-care (difficulty dressing or bathing), and independent living (difficulty doing errands alone). The dataset is public, and it can also be used for obtaining visual results, previewing the dataset and downloading it for further analysis.

  The DHDS system can be assessed online [86], and visualizations and prevalence results depending on the state and health topic can be made with no restrictions. For example, the user can select a state (Arizona) and further select a category (disability estimates), and the results are presented for the overall population and further broken and presented according to several indicators (such as age, sex, ethnicity). The presentation of the results varies, however, depending on the health topic/category. The results can be exported in cvs format or saved as a pdf.

- **FluVaxView**
  This section provides influenza vaccination coverage estimates at the national, regional, and state levels and produces interactive maps, trend lines, bar charts, and data tables. The estimates of influenza coverage are presented for several populations: for persons aged 6 months and older (the general population), healthcare personnel, nursing home residents, and pregnant women. The data for influenza vaccination coverage for the general population were derived from the National Immunization Survey-Flu (NIS-Flu) and the Behavioral Risk Surveillance System (BRFSS). The data for the healthcare personnel were obtained from the National Healthcare Safety Network, those for the nursing residence home were collected from the Long-Term Care Minimum Data Set (MDS) from the Centers for Medicare and Medicaid Services, and those for pregnant women were obtained from the Pregnancy Risk Assessment Monitoring System (PRAMS). The results for vaccination coverage are also presented according to season and population in the form of reports.

Other forms of vaccine coverage estimates are available for children (ChildVaxView), for teenagers (TeenVaxView), for children attending schools (SchoolVaxView), for adults (AdultVaxView), and finally for COVID-19 vaccine uptake (COVIDVaxView). All these online sources have the same aim: to estimate vaccination coverage for these specific populations (and for vaccines against COVID-19) and locate the sports that require additional efforts to increase vaccination coverage. Additionally, depending on the population of interest, the CDC uses different datasets to obtain data related to immunization rates. For example, the COVID-19View relies on data from the following sources: IPSOS KnowledgePanel (an online probability-based survey for those older than 18 years), the National Immunization Survey-Adult COVID-19 Module (NIS-ACM), and the National Immunization Survey-Child COVID-19 Module (NIS-CCM) (both are random-digit dial telephone surveys of US adults and US parents/guardians), NORC AmeriSpeak (an online survey of adult members of the NORC), and the US Census Household Pulse Survey (an online survey investigating the impact of the coronavirus pandemic on households from a social and economic perspective). The other population-specific vaccination coverage tools derive their data from other databases that cover those specific populations. The CDC uses these data for deriving evidence-based decisions to support public health, and the obtained results are presented in the form of reports, journal articles, and easily accessible tools that are also intended for the public.

- **COVID-19 Surveillance**
  The CDC created a publicly available (deidentified) patient-level dataset related to COVID-19 surveillance data [87]. These data are routinely reported to the CDC by public health jurisdictions on the basis of the CSTE Interim Position Statement, which provides definitions for COVID-19 surveillance cases. COVID-19 data are publicly available either as summaries or aggregations of count files (including total counts of cases and deaths by state and by county). By collecting COVID-19-related data, the CDC continuously monitors COVID-19 epidemiological trends, which are inevitable for both preventing and, when necessary, responding to the potential threats caused by this virus.

2.2.5   The World Health Organization Initiatives

The World Health Organization's (WHO's) constitution was enforced on 7 April 1948 and established the first specialized agency of the United Nations [88]. It was intended to make the WHO the world's health champion by merging the best health professionals around the globe, who, by mutual forces, work together to ensure that everyone has an equal chance of leading a safe and healthy life [89]. In a broad sense, the WHO's tasks are aimed at promoting health, keeping the world safe, and serving vulnerable people. Within their mandate, they should perform activities that will enable universal health coverage, protection from health emergencies, and improved health and well-being. To achieve universal health coverage, their tasks are oriented towards improving access to quality primary healthcare services; enabling sustainable financing and financial protection; granting wider access to essential medicines and health products; providing training to the health workforce and advice on labour policies; and improving monitoring, data, and information. In addressing health emergencies, the WHO performs tasks related to preparing for emergencies (identifying, mitigating, and managing risks); preventing emergencies; supporting the development of tools required during outbreaks; detecting and responding to acute health emergencies; and supporting the delivery of essential health services. The tasks associated with addressing health and well-being issues include addressing social determinants, promoting intersectoral approaches for health, and prioritizing health in all policies and healthy settings. Through their work, they aim at preventing noncommunicable diseases, promoting mental health, eliminating antimicrobial resistance, and addressing high-impact communicable diseases. With respect to the WHO's projects that rely on EHD reuse, the following projects are presented below.

- **Global Health Estimates** [90]
  The WHO's Global Health Estimates (GHEs) represent the most up-to-date data related to death and disability at the global level during the period between 2000 and 2019, presented by region and country, age, sex, and cause. Estimates of mortality and morbidity trends are extremely useful tools in making informed decisions on health policy and resource allocation. The GHE data are collected from multiple sources: national vital registration data, latest estimates from WHO technical programmes, United Nations partners and interagency groups, and the Global Burden of Disease and other scientific studies. Some of the WHO's GHEs cover the following health-related indicators: life expectancy; healthy life expectancy; mortality and morbidity; and burden of diseases at the global, regional, and country levels, which are presented depending on age, sex, and cause. Access to and use of GHE data are granted through a range of channels and media, such as the Global Health Observatory [91], which represents an interactive visual summary of global and regional data.
- **Meeting the health SDGs**
  The United Nations Sustainable Development Goals (SDGs), which build on the Millennium Development Goals, refer to 17 goals (and 169 associated targets) agreed upon by all 191 UN Member States that should be achieved by the year 2030. The central role of health is in SDG 3. It includes 13 specific targets that are associated with the WHO's wide spectrum of work. The utilization of the WHO's annual World Health Statistics reports in this case represents a valuable tool that can be used to track and monitor the progress of the WHO's SDG activities to ensure that the activities are aligned with the predefined goals. These reports are the most up-to-date health statistics for the WHO Member States, and they are published annually [92].
- **The Mortality Database and its Use** [93]
  The WHO Mortality Database is composed of mortality data obtained from the national authorities (collected from their civil registration and statistics systems).

Only data with at least 65% completeness are accountable for publication in this database. These annual requests are sent by the WHO to all countries to send their mortality data by cause of death, year, sex, and age since 1950. Today, this database is composed of data from more than 120 countries and areas. The WHO mortality database is used for performing comparative epidemiological studies at the international level. It is also one of the sources of empirical data that are used for producing WHO reports related to SDG health indicators (such as those on noncommunicable diseases and suicides). One example of WHO mortality database use was in 1992, when Peto et al. [94] published a new metric, the smoking impact ratio (SIR), which he used to estimate deaths attributed to tobacco use in developed countries by considering the difference in individual tobacco use. This study revealed that the average loss in life expectancy for those killed by tobacco in middle age (35–69 years) was approximately 23 years, and approximately 20% of people living in developed countries would eventually die due to tobacco consumption. These findings have led to major changes in further tobacco control actions. The WHO's Global Health Estimates (GHE) reports also regularly use data from the WHO mortality database. These GHEs of mortality are published by age, sex, and cause, both at the global level and at the country level.

- **Surveillance-Related Projects.**
  The WHO Outbreak Toolkit site is an online source designed to help epidemiologists and field investigators in situations of complex emergencies and when resources are limited. The existence of regularly updated comprehensive tools can facilitate investigations related to infectious and noninfectious disease outbreaks and hazards. This toolkit should support thorough and detailed outbreak investigations. Its aim is to address the time burden before and during field deployment in researching and identifying important documents and to provide the information necessary to propose an investigation design, define the process of data collection, and formulate response activities. In this way, it can support evaluation of the cause, severity, and risk of extension in a timely manner and facilitate data sharing, collection, and comparability in cases of outbreak investigations. This toolkit was launched in 2017 by the WHO Regional Office for Africa, specifically to support investigations of unknown disease outbreaks [95].
  Global Influenza Surveillance and Response System (GISRS)
  This system has been in use for influenza surveillance at the global level since 1952. To provide protection against influenza, it performs several functions: global surveillance; monitoring of influenza epidemiology and disease; developing mechanisms for preparedness and response to seasonal, pandemic, or zoonotic influenza; and alerting in cases of novel influenza viruses and other respiratory pathogens. GISRS currently comprises institutions located in 129 WHO Member States, such as National Influenza Centers, WHO Collaborating Centres, WHO H5 Reference Laboratories, and WHO Essential Regulatory Laboratories. FluNet is a supportive online tool launched in 1997 that serves for influenza virological surveillance at the global level. These virological data included in FluNet are essential for monitoring the trend of influenza viruses globally and performing epidemiological updates. These country-level data are

publicly available and updated on a weekly basis, and the results are generated as tables, maps, and graphs. The data are collected remotely from National Influenza Centers that are part of the GISRS and from other national influenza reference laboratories that are GISRS collaborators or from WHO regional databases [96].

2.2.6   Organisation for Economic co-Operation and Development (OECD) Initiatives

The OECD is an international organization that connects Member countries with a wide range of partners to work together and tackle ongoing key problems at the global, national, regional, and local levels. They exert their impact through developing standards, programmes, and initiatives. Currently, there are 38 Member countries in the OECD, represented by their ambassadors at the OECD Council, that have a role in defining and overseeing the work of the OECD, as outlined in the OECD Convention. The Member countries can make informed decisions by making use of the data collected by the OECD, collaborating with their experts, with the aim of increasing performance.

The activities of the OECD can be divided into three main areas: informing, influencing, and setting standards. To provide information, the OECD gathers more than 5 billion data points annually and transforms it into knowledge disseminated in reports (more than 500), country surveys, policy briefs, articles, and digital content. This knowledge is also used in informing debates in parliaments, media, and research work, and international policy debates in global forums. They provide data, analytical reports, policy recommendations, and standards for their international collaborators, such as the G20 group, the G7, the Deauville Partnership, Asia Pacific Economic Cooperation (APEC), and the African Union Commission. The OECD exerts its influence by connecting countries and partners around the globe to engage together in bringing new innovative ideas that will help address a range of issues (from inequality, youth unemployment, the gender gap, migrant integration, or ageing in poverty, among others). These issues are addressed by organizing thematic committees, expert and working groups, policy makers and policy shapers where they share insights and ideas to identify the best possible solutions to the current problems. Finally, the OECD sets international standards and codes in collaboration with Member countries. They cover a wide range of standards, from legally binding acts (such as the 1997 Anti-bribery Convention) to recommendations that should guide policy makers regarding best practices in various fields of application. This resulted in over 450 international standards (including conventions, recommendations, guidelines, and declarations) over the past 55 years [97].

The OECD has arranged their activities according to 27 topics, one of which is focused on health-related outcomes (other topics include chemical safety and biosafety, corporate governance, taxes, innovation, industry, and entrepreneurship, among others). They divided their health-related work into several areas: ageing and long-term care, antimicrobial resistance, digital health, the fiscal sustainability of health systems, health data governance, health inequalities and inclusive growth, health expenditure, health system performance assessment, health workforce, mental health, and PaRIS: patient-reported indicator surveys, pharmaceuticals and new technologies, primary care, public health (e.g. obesity, alcohol), quality of care, resilience, and universal health coverage [98]. The selected areas of the OECD's activities where EHD reuse has been applied include the following:

- **Investing in Health System Resilience [99]**
  The COVID-19 pandemic revealed that many health systems are not resilient enough. Resilient health systems are those systems that can respond to critical situations (such as pandemics, economic crises, or the effects of climate change). More specifically, they should be able to address the negative consequences in the most efficient way, obtain a quick recovery, and further adapt to higher performance and preparedness. The OECD invests their efforts in identifying smart and targeted investments in health system resilience that should lead to their improvement and better response to shocks. In their report on the impact of COVID-19 on health systems, they reviewed key issues such as the workforce, digitalization, continuity of care, and mental health (among other topics) and made six recommendations aimed at improving health system resilience and reducing the negative effects of future shocks. Their assessment revealed that health service disruptions resulted in a reduction in diagnostic and surgical procedures in 2020; for example, the number of hip replacements decreased by 16% (compared with 2019) in 31 OECD countries, ranging from 35% (Chile, Costa Rica, and the UK) to less than 5% (in Denmark, Finland, Israel, Latvia, and Switzerland). The data utilized for these analyses were from the OECD Health Statistics, a comprehensive source of data provided from both the OECD and some selected non-OECD countries dating from the 1960s. It collects a wide range of health status data at the population level, including obesity, suicide and life expectancy, healthcare financing/resources, nonmedical determinants of health, expenditures on health, and demographic and economic references, among others [100].

- **Healthcare Quality and Outcomes**
  Patients receiving safe, effective, and adequate healthcare have received public interest among OECD countries, and this objective of health systems has been recognized as the most important. To achieve this goal, assessments and continuous monitoring are needed. The OECD expertise is engaged in this field by assisting assessments of quality of care to help governments identify the strategies that need to be implemented in their health systems that will improve their quality of care.
  One of the projects within this health-related area of OECD work is defining healthcare quality and outcome indicators. In 2021, the OECD performed a data collection process focused on Healthcare Quality and Outcomes (HCQO), which resulted in a total of 64 indicators covering the following topics: primary care, safe prescribing in primary care, acute care, mental healthcare, cancer care,

patient safety, and patient experiences. This collection is based on data from 40 countries, some of which were non-OECD member countries such as Singapore, Malta, and Romania.

The Healthcare Quality and Outcomes programme was previously known as the Healthcare Quality Indicators (HCQI) project and was launched in 2001. Its objective was to identify indicators that can be used to compare healthcare quality at the international level. During the last 20 years, the process of data collection and analysis has been in progress, which has continuously expanded the list of covered dimensions and the number of involved countries [101].

2.2.7 Other Regional Initiatives

2.2.7.1 Health Statistics

HealthStatNSW is the official New South Wales government website, which presents an overview of the statistical information related to NSW population health [102]. The data are collected from many sources, and the statistical outputs are organized such that users can view and download data and select indicators to produce tailored reports covering a wide range of health determinants and outcomes, locations, and specific populations. On the HealthStatNSW website, the data are categorized into different health topics (such as mortality, hospitalizations, overweight, and obesity). For example, "hospitalization" as a health outcome is further categorized alphabetically according to the reasons for hospitalization, e.g. alcohol-attributable hospitalizations, acute myocardial infarction (AMI) hospitalizations, etc. By selecting AMI hospitalizations as an example, the user can retrieve a graphical presentation of the hospitalization rates (which can be presented as numbers or rates per 100,000 people). Comparisons can be made depending on the type of disease and sex. The web presentation also contains technical information about the data that was used for the analyses (in this case, the sources of data were NSW Combined Admitted Patient Epidemiology Data and ABS population estimates [SAPHaRI] and data collected by the Centre for Epidemiology and Evidence, NSW Ministry of Health). It also contains information about the statistical methods that were used, the inclusion/exclusion criteria for the data, and other relevant information.

2.2.7.2 The National Institute for Health and Care Excellence (NICE) Production of Guidance

The NICE operates as an independent, nondepartmental public body that has a role in developing guidelines (in England). In addition to clinical guidelines, they also establish those related to public health, social care, and healthcare. Its aim is to improve the population outcomes of those who are the end users of the NHS and other public health and social care services. The aim of these guidelines is to provide benefits at the population level by considering individual needs and enabling fair distribution of available resources [103].

The NICE provides guidance [104] in the following fields: broad health and social care topics (there are currently 339 guidelines in this field), technology appraisal (which reviews the clinical value and cost effectiveness of new treatments, n = 709), diagnostics (reviews new diagnostic technologies for adoption in the NHS, n = 47), health technology evaluation (aims to explore new ways to support the adoption of health technologies in the NHS, such as early value assessment, n = 11), highly specialized technologies (focus is not reviewing the clinical value and cost effectiveness of specialized treatments, n = 25), interventional procedures (focus is on the efficacy and safety of procedures, n = 589), and medical technologies (reviews new medical devices for adoption in the NHS, n = 65).

The reuse of EHD is very important for the NICE's production of Guidelines. One way in which NICE employs the reuse of health data is by using real-world evidence to inform their guidelines. Examples include:

1. Characterization of health conditions, interventions, healthcare pathways, and patient outcomes and experiences—NICE published highly specialized technology guidance on surgeons performing spinal muscular atrophy treatment by using multiple sources of RWD to describe spinal muscular atrophy.
2. Designing, populating, and validating economic models (such as estimates of resource use, quality of life, event rates, prevalence, incidence, and long-term outcomes), for example, in the case of baseline rates of events, NICE developed a guideline on chronic obstructive pulmonary disease in over 16 s: diagnosis and management reported data from the Clinical Practice Research Datalink GOLD database on baseline chronic obstructive pulmonary disease exacerbation rates by disease severity.
3. Developing or validating digital health technologies (e.g. digital technologies can rely on a clinical algorithm developed using real-world data, and there is a published guideline, "NICE evidence standards framework for digital health technologies").
4. Identifying, characterizing, and addressing health inequalities—for example NICE technology appraisal guidance on the use of crizanlizumab for preventing sickle cell crisis in sickle cell disease patients—generated evidence from the National Haemoglobinopathy Registry and reported a disproportionate burden of sickle cell disease in some minority ethnic groups.
5. Understanding the safety of medical technologies (including medicines, devices, and interventional procedures)—for example, by estimating test accuracy or reproducibility of test results; in the case of biomarkers, NICE published medical technologies guidance on Zio XT for detecting cardiac arrhythmias on the basis of the data obtained from a retrospective observational cohort study.
6. Assessing the impact of interventions (including tests) on service delivery and decisions related to care—NICE diagnostic guidance was published on tumour

profiling tests to support adjuvant chemotherapy decisions in early breast cancer patients by obtaining results from prospective observational studies.
7. Assessing the applicability of clinical trials to patients in the NHS.

2.2.7.3   Australian Institute of Health and Welfare (AIHW) Statistics

The Australian Institute of Health and Welfare (AIHW) is an independent statutory Australian government agency that produces authoritative and accessible information and statistics to inform and support policy and decision makers, with the final goal of achieving better health and well-being at the population level [105]. Some of their specific roles include producing and maintaining standards for statistical information applied in the health, community services, and housing assistance sectors; health and welfare data collection and management (from state, territory, and federal government agencies); performing analyses and disseminating results; and establishing new health and welfare datasets. They collaborate with a wide range of stakeholders, such as the Australian Bureau of Statistics and other Australian government agencies, state and territory governments, local governments, universities, research centres, nongovernment organizations, and international organizations. The Australian Institute of Health and Welfare also collaborates in sharing information with international organizations, including the World Health Organization (WHO) and the Organisation for Economic Co-operation and Development (OECD).

Their health and welfare data include more than 150 datasets related to diverse fields, such as housing assistance, homelessness, perinatal health, disability, cancer, hospitals and hospital activity, alcohol and other drugs, and mortality. Data privacy and confidentiality are maintained and aligned with the requirements of the Privacy Act 1998 (Commonwealth) and the Australian Institute of Health and Welfare Act 1987 (Commowealth). These data are used for producing reports, bulletins, and data products presented on this website (such as dynamic data displays, data cubes, and Tableau products) and are used by the community, policy makers, researchers, and service providers. The contribution of the AIHW in managing population health by collecting and using these diverse datasets can be elaborated in the following case studies relying on data reuse:

- **Putting cancer screening in perspective**

   The report regarding the impact of Australia's cancer screening programmes is a valuable resource that enables the evaluation of their effectiveness. Australia currently has three national screening programmes, and while it first started with ad hoc cervical screening in the 1960s, the first structured screening programmes were introduced in the 1990s. The AIHW published the first national report related to cancer screening programmes in 2018, for which it used data from BreastScreen Australia, the National Cervical Screening Program, the National Bowel Cancer Screening Program, the Australian Cancer Database, the National Death Index, and the National HPV (human papillomavirus) Vaccination

Program Register. The results were encouraging: timely screening lowered the cancer risk in all three cases (breast, cervical, and bowel cancer).

- **Mapping chronic conditions across Australia**

  The interactive online mapping tools developed by AIHWs are regularly used by health professionals to help them improve the services they provide. Since social and economic conditions sometimes affect health and well-being, addressing these issues sometimes requires local solutions. The prevalence of chronic conditions and associated risk factors typically vary on the basis of geographical location, and this information can help healthcare providers know where they should focus and thus prevent and manage them at an earlier stage. In 2021, the AIHW released a series of interactive maps, which were created as a result of combining online geospatial interactive mapping technology with national health data on chronic diseases. As a result, health professionals, policy makers, researchers, and support services can derive customized insights and design evidence-based prevention programmes/strategies and support services aimed at people with chronic conditions (such as diabetes and cardiovascular and kidney disease).

- **Bringing together data on dementia**

  Although Australia was one of the pioneers in developing national dementia policy initiatives in 1992, it lacked a national database that would be utilized for informing and developing policies. Thus, as part of the Australian government's response to this challenge, the AIHW performed the first comprehensive data analyses related to the status of dementia in Australia. This further led to the establishment of the National Centre for Monitoring Dementia (NCMD) in September 2021. The focus of the work of the Centre will be linking administrative data, improving dementia data, and performing analyses of existing linked data.

- **COVID-19 register and linked dataset**

  The AIHW established a COVID-19 register with case data and linked it with other datasets (such as hospital and death data), which enabled researchers to gain new insights into the effects of COVID-19 at the individual, community, and health system levels. The data in this register include administrative and clinical data held by federal, state, and local government agencies, as well as health and welfare service providers. This information (on COVID-19 cases) will be retrieved from the participating states and territories, the Australian Government's National Notifiable Disease Surveillance System, and other administrative data sources.

2.3   Electronic Health Data for Healthcare System Improvement and for Research

The reuse of EHD is particularly relevant for improving healthcare systems and accelerating research. This section elaborates on the aspects of EHD reuse in learning healthcare systems and the benefits associated with utilizing them. It further dives into the field of personalized medicine and explores how different types of real-world data can be integrated with the aim of leveraging unique individual treatments addressing patient needs. One of the few to mention are implementing EHD in pharmacogenomics to determine how patients respond to certain treatments and to what extent information can later be used to tailor personalized care to individuals. The third section covers the utility of EHD for improving the quality and safety of healthcare, for which ample data reveal positive associations, thereby providing space for generating new knowledge that will lead to further improvements. Finally, the last section explores the utilization of EHD for research purposes, whereby it refers to advancing new scientific knowledge and discoveries, such as those involved in drug development, or gaining new understanding of existing or new diseases, among others.

2.3.1   Learning Healthcare Systems

According to the Institute of Medicine's original definition, a Learning Health System (LHS) is a more comprehensive system where "science, informatics, incentives, and culture are aligned for continuous improvement and innovation, with best practices seamlessly embedded in the delivery process and new knowledge captured as an integral byproduct of the delivery experience" [106].

With the emergence of personalized medicine, the aim of healthcare facilities that can move a leap forward from standardized care to personalized medicine has become necessary. For this process to take place, a transformation from a healthcare approach based mainly on evidence-based medicine to a healthcare approach complemented by the potential of data collected in daily clinical practice in the form of EHR and united with patient-reported measures is needed, not only to contribute to personalized care but also to improve the accuracy of current prediction models and enhance the decision-making process of clinicians.

LHS may be one of the manifestations of this process, as it is able to generate and apply the best evidence for the collaborative healthcare choices of each patient and provider, thus ensuring innovation, quality, safety, and value in healthcare, with personalization of healthcare being one of the aims of LHS [107]. On the other hand, among the benefits achieved for patients are (1) better evidence-based care as a result of benchmarking, (2) tracking of outcomes available at the point of care, (3) the possibility of self-management by patients, (4) health optimization as a result of collaborative visualization of the patient's condition, and (5) value found from the patient's perspective as a result of the patient's knowledge about the patient's condition [108]. Examples focusing on LHS and EHD reuse are described in the following paragraphs.

- **Retrospective Use of EHD as Part of LHS:** As much as LHS allows better targeting of the right treatments and interventions to the right patients, they also leverage the opportunity to use routine data as a source of information, thus providing special support in areas such as drug safety. In this case, LHS supports the transition from the traditional paradigm of randomized controlled trials (RCTs), which are the standard for demonstrating the efficacy and safety of drugs, implying high financial and operational costs, to the use of retrospective information from EHRs as a source of shared data and answers. More generally, examples of this process already exist, and the milestones achieved thus far can be seen with the results obtained from Kaiser Permanente and its integrated EHR system, which, in conjunction with big data analytics, has improved health outcomes in sectors such as maternal and neonatal care [109].

- **Supporting Drug Research:** There are also results showing the potential of these innovations. In the case of the Ongoing Telmisartan Alone and in Combination with Ramipril Global Endpoint Trial (ONTARGET), the results of retrospective research using EHR data and mirroring the patient selection criteria of the RCT were able to obtain "almost identical" results, which took only 12 weeks, instead of 7 years to perform, and costs less than a hundredth of the trial, which cost tens of millions of dollars [110].

- **Other Multiple Opportunities for Retrospective Data:** As more data are becoming electronic, very large repositories of data are therefore allowing retrospective cohort analysis to become common. This finding supports the application of retrospective cohort studies for patient stratification, a key step in providing personalized care to construct a customized treatment plan for each patient group. Organizations such as IBM have already captured the value of these data through the application of machine learning, data mining, and data visualization techniques, which are needed to leverage large amounts of data into consumable and relevant information [111]. One example of such a tool is CareFlow, for which physicians can visualize care pathways for patients using information from similar patient pathways, thus providing information to the physician on which pathways were successful and lead to health improvements and which do not [112]. CareFlow aims to harness the extensive longitudinal data available in electronic medical records (EMRs) and thus provide clinicians with a powerful, data-driven tool for designing personalized care plans. By analysing patients' relevant clinical data, CareFlow uses patient similarity analytics to identify and compare individuals with similar clinical profiles from EMRs, aiding in the development of tailored treatment strategies.

This tool, together with other tools derived from patient similarity metric (PSM) learning, has proven useful, especially in data-rich contexts such as intensive care units (ICUs), where the prediction of a minimum adverse condition on the basis of patient behaviour can provide important support to physicians. Additionally, the component of patient similarity analytics could also be able to predict if the patient is going to experience a medical event within a specific time horizon, thus providing highly valuable insights to physicians in a way that would be very difficult to provide otherwise [111].

2.3.2   Personalized Medicine

Throughout most of the medical history, a wide approach to diagnosis and treatment has been used. With the realization of human genome sequencing in 1990, a shift in this system of care began to take shape. This significant event also coincided with the rise of the term "personalized medicine", which sought to offer a more individualized approach to patient care [113, 114]. This goal could be attained in part by supporting the linking of patients' genomic and clinical profiles, which enables a deeper understanding of disease and the development of more effective treatments.

Today, the availability of large amounts of data, as well as the emergence of genomic data health systems and repositories, is opening new avenues for the management of health for individuals. For example, projects such as the HapMap Project have leveraged this potential to create catalogues of human genetic variations shared across many individuals, thus resulting in the first generation of microarrays that assayed hundreds of thousands of genetic variants in a single test [115]. HapMap is an effective tool for investigating the genetic elements that contribute to other components, such as environmental factors, as well as the efficacy of and unfavourable reactions to medications and vaccinations, in addition to its utility for analysing the relationship between genetic profiles and disease [116]. Some other examples of reuse are reported herein.

- **Wearable Sensor Data Coupled with EHD for Disease Monitoring and Prediction:** The ability of sensors to capture and interpret real-time data presents a chance to combat prevalent chronic diseases that can be prevented. As an illustration, studies using Bluetooth low-energy (BLE) sensors in combination with machine learning-based algorithms have demonstrated the potential to collect and manage real-time data on various parameters, including blood glucose, effectively monitor the vital signs of diabetic patients, and provide early diabetes disease prediction given the user's sensors [117]. The potential of these technologies in conjunction with EHD could not only detect the incidence of diseases at a wider scale and lower cost but also use real-time data processing to offer personalized lifestyle recommendations, as could be the case with diet and physical activity, thereby providing patients with an opportunity to track and improve their health status, preventing critical conditions in the future [117].
- **Home Monitoring as a Support Measure for Personalized Care in the Clinical Setting:** The outcomes of chronic and other diseases may be impacted by timely patient–provider communication that uses decision support tools to individualize care. In fact, a 6-month study on the effects of home blood pressure

(BP) and systolic blood pressure (SBP) monitoring, for instance, revealed that patients with higher home BP upload frequencies had noticeably higher probabilities of reaching home BP targets. Additionally, 55.9% of the participants met their office BP goals by the programme's conclusion. Along with increasing their diet of fruits and vegetables, patients also made other improvements to their way of life, such as consuming fewer items rich in fat and salt. These findings point to the possibility of home monitoring and the systematic use of data supplied by patients to produce individualized care plans that support and facilitate efficient clinical management [118].

- **Patient Similarity Metrics for Improved Prediction Performance:** As clinical outcome predictions based on one-size-fits-all models tend to offer suboptimal performance for individual patients with unique characteristics, the use of patient similarity metrics (PSMs), which are analogous to personalized product recommendations in e-commerce, could provide multiple solutions, especially in data-intensive and critical decision support scenarios, as is the case in ICUs. In a related study, clinical data from the first day of ICU admission were analysed. An analysis of data collected from 17,152 adults revealed that the use of data from a small subset of patients and therefore the analysis of only similar patients resulted in improved performance. In addition to the increased computational burden, big data technologies could help facilitate this process [119].
- **Pharmacogenomic Implementation:** The use of information to predict the response of patients to a specific drug has been one of the earliest successful demonstrations of EHD-driven personalized medicine. As evidence has demonstrated the potential of genetics to alter the pharmacodynamics of a drug, including absorption, distribution, metabolism, or elimination [120], pharmacogenomics (PGx) offers the possibility of identifying drug responders and nonresponders; preventing or avoiding adverse events; and optimizing drug response [115]. Initiatives in this field have already demonstrated success, with examples such as the US-based Pharmacogenomics Research Network serving as a catalyst to support PGx discoveries. Currently, although fewer than 10% of published genome-wide association studies have focused on Pgx, there are already over 200 drugs that have included information on their FDA-approved labels, sharing information on specific actions to be taken on the basis of the genetic profile or variants of users. Additionally, we anticipate that genomic applications of personalized medicine, including PGx and preventive health, will scale widely in many health systems, as billions of dollars in worldwide expenditures are being made to integrate genetics into healthcare [115].

2.3.3 Healthcare Quality and Safety

There is ample empirical evidence on the relationship between EHRs and healthcare quality. In addition, the impact of decision support systems on quality is still supported by mixed evidence, with more recent evidence revealing a more significant impact than previous evidence did. Among the evidence available, more recent research provides stronger support for the notion that EHD or EHRs improve quality, with some researchers finding that >60% of studies find a positive consequence from the implementation of EHR systems. Among the beneficial effects, EHRs can provide beneficial effects in preventive care for a variety of conditions and can also provide decision support via algorithms in combination with surveillance technology, significantly reducing sepsis mortality. Other improvements include prescription errors, even in the absence of support systems, as well as other safety gains related to mortality reduction, especially in high-severity patients [121].

Other studies have shown that EHR interoperability positively influences variables such as medication safety and reduces patient safety events and costs. However, a study carried out by Romano and Stafford reported no consistent associations, with only 1 of 20 indicators showing significantly better performance when the associations among EHR implementation, clinical decision support (CDS), and quality improvement were investigated [122]. In the case of quality and safety of care, the benefits of EHR remain unclear, among other causes, due to the large heterogeneity of interventions, designs, and outcome measures regarding EHR evaluation [123]. Some specific EHD reuse applications to improve safety and quality of care are provided below.

- **EHD Reuse for Improving Paediatric Care:** For highly specific areas of healthcare, such as paediatric treatment, EHRs may also help improve quality. Most inpatient quality measures do not apply to children, who represent a substantial group. On the basis of their overall value for efforts to improve quality, research has nominated 18 indicators for inclusion in the paediatric quality indicator collection. In the case of paediatric indicators, validity specific to children is needed, and this must be emphasized. These new indicators might help prioritize efforts for quality improvement at the local and national levels, among other advantages [124].
- **Improving Patient Care by Providing Individual Feedback:** One example is the Anaesthesiology Performance Improvement and Reporting Exchange (ASPIRE), which is a quality and patient safety initiative that aims to enhance patient care by anaesthesia providers with personalized feedback. As part of this process, and on the basis of previously established priorities, each participating site can develop tailored safety goals together with a selection of quality measures. The individual providers subsequently receive monthly emails with information about their performance and how it compares to the department average. Additionally, further potential for quality improvement may be found by accounting for risk variables on the basis of the patient mix of each individual practitioner. As part of the current milestones of the initiative, preventing hypotension in patients undergoing noncardiac surgery, regardless of other risk factors, is one of the ASPIRE procedures currently in place [125, 126].

2.3.4 Supporting Research Activities

Reusing EHD for research purposes refers to applying these data to accelerate the generation of new knowledge and insights related to healthcare, such as accelerating drug discoveries, finding new applications of existing drugs, and discovering new pathways in disease progression. As natural language processing (NLP)[2] methods increase in popularity, the utilization of future technologies for the processing of data that could ultimately eliminate manual entry could also significantly increase the amount of available data for research purposes. Although the majority of EHRs were not designed with the intention of using information for research purposes, converting existing EHR information into a format that can be used for analysis is possible, although it is resource-intensive. NLP could transform this as having the potential to transform clinical data into analysable data elements, thus turning Big Data into smart data [127]. Moreover, current proof-of-concepts using NLP to mine EHR data for research purposes have proven this technology to be successful in tasks such as extracting cancer stage information, creating oncology treatment summaries, and automating the determination of prostate cancer risk groups [128]. Examples of the successful use of NLP to access data already exist. This is the case for the case register interactive search (CRIS) system, which contains the clinical records of more than 250,000 patients, including the majority of its information in free text form [129, 130]. Through recent advances in natural language processing, the data are now available for large-scale research, which has led to over 50 publications using the dataset, including the opportunity to perform research on heard-to-reach populations such as homeless individuals, people suffering from mental diseases such as bipolar disorders, and others [131–134].

Nevertheless, AI has also been applied to imaging and other types of health data, which provides a promising outlook. Current examples of the potential of this technology have been described in the field of ophthalmology, for which the volume of data has grown particularly fast. Among the conditions for which the technology has already been applied are diabetic retinopathy, age-related macular degeneration, and cataracts. The results have also been promising, with acute angle closure glaucoma obtaining moderate performance (67%) in the prediction of the risk of progression to surgical intervention in patients suffering from open-angle glaucoma, as well as 88% success in acute angle closure glaucoma diagnosis via supervised machine learning techniques [135]. Some other examples of EHD reuse for advancing new knowledge are presented below.

---

[2] Natural language processing (NLP) is a branch of artificial intelligence and computer science focused on enabling machines to comprehend, interpret, and interact using human languages. By combining rule-based computational linguistics with statistical methods, machine learning, and deep learning techniques, NLP allows digital systems to process, understand, and even generate text and spoken language. It facilitates the interpretation of human communication by leveraging machine learning models trained on vast language datasets, bridging the gap between human language and computer understanding (https://www.ibm.com/topics/natural-language-processing).

- **Research Potential of EHD from Administrative Databases:** When biobanks are linked to administrative databases, various data sources, such as genomic, physiological, and self-reported data, can be connected with hospital episodes and death registration, creating powerful tools for information retrieval about risks and protective factors for various diseases. As an example of the impact of similar approaches, the UK Biobank collects 500,000 individuals from 40–69 years of age and linked data from multiple sources, including hospital episode characteristics in England, as well as comparable datasets in other countries, such as Scotland and Wales. The datasets included administrative data from hospitals, including physical and mental health admissions as well as ICD-10 diagnosis codes. These data provide an opportunity to enrich biobank data in a cost-effective manner as well as to identify cases of psychiatric diseases [136].
- **Supporting Drug Discoveries—Drug Repurposing:** One study explored the feasibility of leveraging EHRs and automated informatics techniques to validate the recent finding that metformin use is associated with reduced cancer mortality, thereby examining its potential for drug repurposing. They integrated two extensive EHR systems from Vanderbilt University Medical Center and Mayo Clinic with their respective tumour registries and formed a cohort of 32,415 cancer patients at Vanderbilt and 79,258 cancer patients from Mayo between 1995 and 2010. They further applied automated informatics methods to identify individuals with type 2 diabetes within this cancer cohort and to collect data on their drug exposure, along with other relevant covariates such as smoking status. EHR data indicated that metformin use was linked to reduced mortality following a cancer diagnosis compared with diabetic and nondiabetic cancer patients not using metformin. These results suggest the potential of metformin as a chemotherapeutic drug, and this study serves as an example of how EHR data can be utilized for cost effective and thorough validation of drug-repurposing signals [137]. Another recent example occurred early in the COVID-19 pandemic, when omic data were used to identify common molecular factors involved in host–coronavirus interactions, including those involved in the COVID-19 and Middle East respiratory syndrome-CoV outbreaks [138]. These discoveries were then connected with real-world data from claims and genetic sources to identify two existing medications that could be repurposed to reduce viral replication and enhance patient outcomes. Additionally, at the 2021 American Society for Clinical Oncology (ASCO) meeting, researchers compared more than 325,000 tumour samples with more than 28,000 matched plasma samples to detect kinase fusions, revealing a high level of agreement between fusion events in tumours and novel liquid biopsy samples [139].
- **Supporting Drug Discoveries—Identifying New Biomarkers:** EHD can be used for validating and identifying novel biomarkers that can aid in the development of new treatments, such as in the case of cancer. One research group developed a computational tool named Zodiac, which was designed to merge existing knowledge on cancer genetic interactions with new information provided by The Cancer Genome Atlas (TCGA) data. It can be utilized to investigate new gene–

gene interactions, transcriptional regulation, and various other molecular interactions in cancer [140].

- **Supporting Drug Discoveries—Identifying Novel Disease Relationships:** When combined with molecular and genetic data, population-based disease relationships and comorbidities can help uncover the mechanisms behind complex diseases and identify new treatments. Exploring relationships within a disease network can reveal common pathophysiological mechanisms, offering new insights into disease aetiology and revealing potential drug targets. Moreover, if a compound is effective for one disease within a disease cluster, it might be applicable to other diseases within the same cluster. EHR databases are valuable resources for systematically mapping disease relationships, understanding disease progression, and analysing directionality. The integration of data mining from EHR databases with network analysis has shown considerable promise [141]. For example, Hanauer et al. [142] also utilized EHR data and focused on analysing free-text clinical problem summary lists from 1.5 million entries across 327,000 patients at the University of Michigan. They employed a tool called Molecular Concept Map to compute odds ratios and P values for each pair of diagnostic associations. This approach allowed them to confirm disease relationships that were known and discover new relationships, some of which were later confirmed in the literature. For example, they identified a novel association between granuloma annulare and osteoarthritis. Both conditions can be treated with niacin [143, 144], suggesting that they may share a common biological pathway and potentially overlapping drug targets.

2.4   Electronic Health Data for the Artificial Intelligence Market

Artificial intelligence (AI) technologies and electronic health data (EHD) reuse are transforming healthcare by enabling more precise, data-driven insights. Through advanced algorithms, AI can analyse vast amounts of EHD—such as the previously mentioned EHRs and genetic information—to discover new patterns, predict patient outcomes, and identify potential drug-repurposing opportunities. This approach enhances disease diagnosis, treatment personalization, and the discovery of novel therapeutic targets. By integrating AI with EHD, healthcare systems can improve decision-making, reduce costs, and accelerate the development of new treatments, ultimately leading to better patient care and outcomes. This subparagraph briefly presents some of the major applications of EHD reuse in developing AI tools and algorithms that have been applied in healthcare.

2.4.1   The Application of Artificial Intelligence in Healthcare

With the rapid surge of AI technologies now being part of daily life for common technologies, including the internet, transportation, and others, its broad application in healthcare is a matter of time. Therefore, applications of AI in healthcare have already taken place at a certain scale, with AI technologies providing promising potential opportunities for providing patients with personalized healthcare recommendations, generating virtual care programmes for chronic diseases and other health conditions, informing population health management, improving clinical trial participation, and others. Below, there are some current general uses of AI in healthcare.

- **Administrative Costs and Burden Reduction:** NLP and other tools could reduce and eliminate the burden of different administrative tasks. Organizations such as Amazon Web Services are already working on these potential applications, thus using NLP to extract and interpret handwritten notes and other information from medical records. Other large public organizations, such as Medicare, are also capitalizing and finding results from these technologies. In the latter case, the Centers for Medicare and Medicaid Services (CMS), after finding that >8% of their payments were improper, started to employ a testing methodology denominated comprehensive error rate testing (CERT), which uses AI to predict fraudulent or improper payments, a technology that has saved them already $42 billion in the process [145].
- **Expanding Access for Rural and Hard-to-Reach Populations:** Implementing AI-related technologies such as chatbots and voice assistants could reduce the resources needed to support rural or hard-to-reach populations, offering solutions to provide information to doctors without needing to be personally available, thus increasing the possibility of asynchronous and virtual care. This could represent a major opportunity not only for those living in rural areas but also for all populations that, owing to a lack of resources of different means (financial, transportation, available time, etc.), could benefit from obtaining this type of care [145].
- **Augmented Intelligence Use for Healthcare:** With respect to the use of AI in healthcare, it is important to note that specialists have highlighted that the goal of AI use would not be to replace the physician's judgement but rather to support a process that could be defined as "augmented intelligence"; this would mean that the physician's judgement would therefore be supported in their decision by the use of technology rather than being replaced, offering the physician the opportunity to prioritize patient symptoms and assess a range of diagnostic possibilities quickly, for example [145].

Importantly, the extended use of these potential applications will therefore require an action plan to achieve the full potential of AI in the coming years. As an example and among the recommendations to support this use of AI for actionable opportunities, the "February 2019 Executive Order on Maintaining American

Leadership in Artificial Intelligence" has developed a set of objectives that could be replicated or used as a framework to increase the potential of AI in healthcare, summarized as follows: (1) promoting sustained investment in AI, (2) enhancing access to high and fully traceable data, (3) reducing barriers to the use of AI technologies, (4) ensuring that technical standards to minimize vulnerability, (5) training the next generation, and (6) developing and implementing an action plan.

2.4.2   Use of Electronic Health Data to Train and Develop Algorithms

With an increase in chronic diseases such as type 2 diabetes affecting both high- and middle- to low-income countries, the development of tools that treat these diseases from a preventive standpoint has become necessary. In the era of technology and digital data, a potential application to address such issues is the linkage between algorithms and EHD. Examples of this potential have already been reported for preventable diseases such as type 2 diabetes, which has achieved high results in terms of sensitivity (95%) and specificity (87%) in different populations, including paediatric populations [146].

The use of algorithms therefore proposes future opportunities in different areas, including the identification of major structural birth defects via automated healthcare data to assess maternal vaccine safety [147] and the low-cost access of clinical data for cancer prognosis [148]. This use that merges administrative or other health data with algorithm applications may also be particularly useful for the identification and support of populations experiencing inadequate care, as may be the case, for example, for people with intellectual and development disabilities, therefore facilitating the planning of specialized treatment or support programmes [149]. Additionally, with financial resources always scarce, including in the public health field, some research has shown promising results in the use of machine learning-based models that are not only able to predict diseases such as type 2 diabetes with a further anticipation of 5 years but also able to reduce healthcare costs after, for example, locating the top 5% of patients at high risk, which ultimately could represent >25% of the annual diabetes costs. This level of information and analysis brought by the potential use of algorithms broadly in healthcare could therefore shape new opportunities for decision-making for population health planning and prevention programmes [150].

However, the application of EHD for these purposes is not without limitations. With commercial insurance data missing at least half of their data on demographics such as ethnicity or language, there is a concern that models developed to be applied when more data are included could provide inaccurate analyses as a result. A similar concern applies to algorithms that may have been developed for specific populations (i.e. younger people, white people, etc.) and that may not be applicable to other more marginalized populations, i.e. patients attending community hospitals.

This, among other issues, could not only hinder the wide application of algorithms but also contribute in some manner to worsening social or economic disparities. Although machine learning techniques that have been developed to account for this missing data could provide a solution to this problem, it is important to note that current developed techniques may not be used consistently. A similar case could take place with populations experiencing a low sample size, a current issue with other types of tools, such as RCTs and clinical studies. A small sample size could therefore be misinterpreted because the machine learning clinical decision support system was developed with larger population sizes in mind, thus leading to inaccurate prediction models for these groups as well [151]. Some additional examples of EHD reuse are presented in the following paragraphs.

- **Logistic regression-based algorithms:** A tool with several uses for a variety of disorders and diseases across the health spectrum is provided by EHD in conjunction with logistic regression algorithms, with research demonstrating the effectiveness of logistic regression algorithms when applied to colonoscopy to distinguish clearly between screening and other purpose colonoscopes to better understand associated parameters, including screening uptake, adherence, results, and others. The least absolute shrinkage and selection operator (LASSO)-based techniques used to create the model yielded a sensitivity and specificity of 0.88 and 0.90, respectively [152]. Other similar algorithms have also been used to identify patients with nontraumatic spinal cord dysfunctions [153], as well as depression, which is the leading cause of disability worldwide, with the highest performance (AUC, 0.77), followed by deep learning algorithms (AUC, 0.74) [154].
- **Hierarchical Algorithms:** Research has demonstrated the effectiveness of using hierarchical algorithms for the definition of cirrhosis aetiology using routinely collected healthcare data, achieving a sensitivity/positive predictive value (PPV) >75% and specificity/negative predictive value (NPV) >90% [155].
- **Testing algorithms by using EHD data:** Some models have used EHD to develop and test algorithms for patient identification purposes. This is the case for an algorithm that was selected after running a test on 5000 of it for the identification of patients suffering from inflammatory bowel disease (IBD). After running the test in contrast with patient cohort registries, the authors identified an algorithm that could achieve a sensitivity of 76.8% with a specificity of 96.2%, which achieved the result by identifying patients between 18 and 64 years of age who had registered 5 physician contacts or hospitalizations within 4 years and even finding better results for patients >65 years of age who had also registered a pharmacy claim for an IBD-related medication [156].
- **Convolutional Neural Network (CNN) Algorithms:** Because the lack of data is one main challenge in the use of algorithms and machine learning techniques for multiple purposes, some algorithms are being developed to address this challenge, thereby offering new opportunities for disease analysis when a lack of data remains or is consistent. This is the case for the CNN algorithm, which uses structured and unstructured hospital data and a latent factor model to reconstruct

the missing information, thus achieving a 94.8% convergence speed, which is faster than that of previous CNN-based unimodal disease risk prediction algorithms.

- **EHD is used for nonintrusive population assessment:** An additional benefit that could be derived from the use of EHD from populations is that it permits researchers to be able to produce results and conclusions from patients' data without further affecting the daily lives of the subjects of study. Therefore, as analysis technologies and algorithms improve, information that is collected as part of a care process becomes even more useful and is therefore able to be used for research, thus saving patients time and reducing the friction of data collection without sacrificing the potential uses of data. For example, a retrospective cohort study on data from the Kuwait Health Network (KHN) allowed Farran et al. to classify patients suffering from diabetes and hypertension with accuracies of >85% for diabetes and > 90% for hypertension, using simple nonlaboratory-based parameters, and even finding better performance when ethnic-specific and combined models were applied [157].

- **At-risk group identification for early prevention programmes:** With the advancement of machine learning algorithms, there is a useful addition to logistic regression models that could therefore support the planning and implementation of early prevention programmes for at-risk groups, as the models predict population outcomes that could be prevented, therefore not only collaborating on the identification of potential outcomes but also serving to identify such populations to implement highly focused early prevention programmes at a reduced cost [158]. Research evidence has proven the theoretical effectiveness of these machine learning algorithms in preventing conditions such as acute kidney injury (AKI), as they are able to predict the likelihood of patients suffering from AKI within 24, 48, and 72 hours of anticipation of the event via information from data collected at wards, thus allowing clinicians to intervene before organ damage starts to appear [159].

- **Algorithm uses for telemedicine**: With the increased use of telemedicine applications to support different populations, including the increasing elderly population, the development of algorithms to support this process provides an opportunity to further enhance remote care, thus increasing the autonomy level and quality of life of patients. This is the case for the gradient boost decision tree (GBDT), which has proven to be the best method for the prediction of blood pressure in multiple individuals, increasing its prediction performance as demographic and other data are added [160].

- **Deep learning for latent patient classification**: Deep learning has been used in medicine for tasks like brain circuit reconstruction and drug activity prediction, but not for general-purpose patient representations from EHRs. Recent advances applied stacked denoising autoencoders (SDAs) to large-scale EHR data, creating "deep patient" representations for broad clinical applications, unlike prior task-specific models. The method was evaluated by predicting diverse future diseases, demonstrating its versatility across clinical domains. By creating a representation of the patient through all their data (lab tests, medications, diagnosis, procedures, etc.), it is now possible to automatize personalized prescriptions, treatment recommendations, and clinical trial recruitment [161].

- **Natural Language Processing and uses on EHR data**: Natural language processing (NLP) plays a significant role in deriving clinical insights from electronic health records. However, its potential is constrained by challenges such as limited annotated datasets and insufficient automated tools. Recent advances have highlighted its many uses regarding risk prediction; some examples include:

  - **Suicide attempt detection:** Identifying first-time suicide attempts is challenging due to limited data, reliance on self-reports, and patients concealing suicidal thoughts. Researchers have explored using EHR data with NLP and machine learning for detection. One study [162] used cTAKES to extract clinical outcomes from medical notes, requiring no preprocessing, identifying concepts, and allowing to test models like Random Forest and LASSO. Another study [163] employed Invenio, an NLP tool built on cTAKES, to analyse EHR text for adolescent suicide risk, leveraging features like entity recognition and cross-validation. Both approaches showed promise but highlighted the need for further refinement and benchmarking, and comparison with gold standard techniques. Still, the potential to improve early detection of suicide risk, enable personalized interventions, and enhance mental healthcare remains.
  - **Automated HIV risk assessment:** Feller et al. [164] developed an automated system for assessing HIV risk using EHRs, aiming to overcome limitations in capturing important behavioural and social factors from structured medical text. Their method utilizes machine learning and NLP to analyse unstructured data, such as information on sexual orientation and activity, which are essential for accurate HIV risk detection. By processing clinical notes, the system identifies key terms, analyses underlying topics, and selects relevant features to predict individuals at high risk, providing a more complete and automated approach to risk assessment.
  - **Diagnosing lupus nephritis:** Lupus nephritis is difficult to diagnose because critical data, such as kidney biopsy histology notes, are embedded in unstructured text. To tackle this, Deng et al. [165] created an NLP-based system to analyse clinical notes for early detection of nephritis. Using inpatient and outpatient datasets, they tested a rule-based algorithm alongside three NLP models built on logistic regression with unique feature sets. Despite improving identification of lupus nephritis and enhancing lupus insights, the method's accuracy was hindered by missing lab results and a limited sample size.

References

1. World Health Organization (2022) Sharing and reuse of health-related data for research purposes: WHO policy and implementation guidance. https://www.who.int/publications/i/item/9789240044968. Accessed 25 Sep 2024

2. Galea S, Tracy M (2007) Participation rates in epidemiologic studies. Ann Epidemiol 17:643–653. https://doi.org/10.1016/j.annepidem.2007.03.013

3. Jensen PB, Jensen LJ, Brunak S (2012) Mining electronic health records: towards better research applications and clinical care. Nat Rev Genet 13:395–405. https://doi.org/10.1038/nrg3208

4. Durojaiye AB, Puett LL, Levin S et al (2018) Linking electronic health record and trauma registry data: assessing the value of probabilistic linkage. Methods Inf Med 57:261–269. https://doi.org/10.1055/S-0039-1681087/ID/JR180048-12/BIB

5. Nichol ST, Spiropoulou CF, Morzunov S et al (1993) Genetic identification of a hantavirus associated with an outbreak of acute respiratory illness. Science 262:914–917. https://doi.org/10.1126/SCIENCE.8235615

6. Holmes EC, Zhang LQ, Robertson P et al (1995) The molecular epidemiology of human immunodeficiency virus type 1 in Edinburgh. J Infect Dis 171:45–53. https://doi.org/10.1093/INFDIS/171.1.45

7. Popovich KJ, Snitkin ES (2017) Whole genome sequencing-implications for infection prevention and outbreak investigations. Curr Infect Dis Rep 19:15. https://doi.org/10.1007/S11908-017-0570-0

8. Joensen KG, Scheutz F, Lund O et al (2014) Real-time whole-genome sequencing for routine typing, surveillance, and outbreak detection of verotoxigenic *Escherichia coli*. J Clin Microbiol 52:1501–1510. https://doi.org/10.1128/JCM.03617-13

9. Graham RMA, Doyle CJ, Jennison AV (2014) Real-time investigation of a *Legionella pneumophila* outbreak using whole-genome sequencing. Epidemiol Infect 142:2347–2351. https://doi.org/10.1017/S0950268814000375

10. Inns T, Lane C, Peters T et al (2015) A multicountry Salmonella Enteritidis phage type 14b outbreak associated with eggs from a German producer: "near real-time" application of whole-genome sequencing and food chain investigations, United Kingdom, May to September 2014. Euro Surveill 20:21098. https://doi.org/10.2807/1560-7917.ES2015.20.16.21098

11. Cook R, Karesh W, Osofsky S (2004) Conference Summary One World, One Health: building interdisciplinary bridges to health in a globalized world. https://www.oneworldonehealth.org/sept2004/owoh_sept04.html. Accessed 25 Sep 2024

12. Trewby H, Nadin-Davis SA, Real LA, Biek R (2017) Processes underlying rabies virus incursions across US–Canada border as revealed by whole-genome Phylogeography. Emerg Infect Dis 23:1454–1461. https://doi.org/10.3201/EID2309.170325

13. Filejski C (2016) Rabies: the changing face of rabies in Canada. Can Commun Dis Rep 42:118–120. https://doi.org/10.14745/CCDR.V42I06A01

14. Kamath PL, Foster JT, Drees KP et al (2016) Genomics reveals historic and contemporary transmission dynamics of a bacterial disease among wildlife and livestock. Nat Commun 7:11448. https://doi.org/10.1038/NCOMMS11448

15. Godfroid J (2017) Brucellosis in livestock and wildlife: zoonotic diseases without pandemic potential in need of innovative one health approaches. Arch Public Health 75:34. https://doi.org/10.1186/S13690-017-0207-7

16. Gardy JL, Loman NJ (2018) Towards a genomics-informed, real-time, global pathogen surveillance system. Nat Rev Genet 19:9–20. https://doi.org/10.1038/NRG.2017.88

17. Croen LA, Grether JK, Yoshida CK et al (2005) Maternal autoimmune diseases, asthma and allergies, and childhood autism spectrum disorders: a case–control study. Arch Pediatr Adolesc Med 159:151–157. https://doi.org/10.1001/archpedi.159.2.151

18. Croen LA, Yoshida CK, Odouli R, Newman TB (2005) Neonatal hyperbilirubinemia and risk of autism spectrum disorders. Pediatrics 115:e135–e138. https://doi.org/10.1542/PEDS.2004-1870

19. Musser ED, Hawkey E, Kachan-Liu SS et al (2014) Shared familial transmission of autism spectrum and attention-deficit/hyperactivity disorders. J Child Psychol Psychiatry 55:819–827. https://doi.org/10.1111/JCPP.12201

20. Armstrong-Wells J, Johnston SC, Wu YW et al (2009) Prevalence and predictors of perinatal hemorrhagic stroke: results from the Kaiser pediatric stroke study. Pediatrics 123:823–828. https://doi.org/10.1542/PEDS.2008-0874

21. Moorman AC, Gordon SC, Rupp LB et al (2013) Baseline characteristics and mortality among people in care for chronic viral hepatitis: the chronic hepatitis cohort study. Clin Infect Dis 56:40–50. https://doi.org/10.1093/CID/CIS815

22. Kanaya AM, Adler N, Moffet HH et al (2011) Heterogeneity of diabetes outcomes among Asians and Pacific islanders in the U.S. Diabetes Care 34:930–937. https://doi.org/10.2337/dc10-1964

23. Laraia BA, Karter AJ, Warton EM et al (2012) Place matters: neighborhood deprivation and cardiometabolic risk factors in the Diabetes Study of Northern California (DISTANCE). Soc Sci Med 74:1082–1090. https://doi.org/10.1016/j.socscimed.2011.11.036

24. Selby JV (1997) Linking automated databases for research in managed care settings. Ann Intern Med 127:719. https://doi.org/10.7326/0003-4819-127-8_Part_2-199710151-00056

25. Hibbard JU, Wilkins I, Sun L et al (2010) Respiratory morbidity in late preterm births. JAMA 304:419–425. https://doi.org/10.1001/JAMA.2010.1015

26. Männistö T, Mendola P, Liu D et al (2015) Acute air pollution exposure and blood pressure at delivery among women with and without hypertension. Am J Hypertens 28:58–72. https://doi.org/10.1093/AJH/HPU077

27. Mendola P, Mumford SL, Männistö TI et al (2015) Controlled direct effects of preeclampsia on neonatal health after accounting for mediation by preterm birth. Epidemiology 26:17–26. https://doi.org/10.1097/EDE.0000000000000213

28. Robledo CA, Mendola P, Yeung E et al (2015) Preconception and early pregnancy air pollution exposures and risk of gestational diabetes mellitus. Environ Res 137:316–322. https://doi.org/10.1016/J.ENVRES.2014.12.020

29. Qizilbash N, Gregson J, Johnson ME et al (2015) BMI and risk of dementia in two million people over two decades: a retrospective cohort study. Lancet Diabetes Endocrinol 3:431–436. https://doi.org/10.1016/S2213-8587(15)00033-9

30. Dhalwani NN, West J, Sultan AA et al (2014) Women with celiac disease present with fertility problems no more often than women in the general population. Gastroenterology 147:1267–1274.e1. https://doi.org/10.1053/J.GASTRO.2014.08.025

31. Mukamal KJ, Wellenius GA, Suh HH, Mittleman MA (2009) Weather and air pollution as triggers of severe headaches. Neurology 72:922–927. https://doi.org/10.1212/01.wnl.0000344152.56020.94

32. May L, Carim M, Yadav K (2011) Adult asthma exacerbations and environmental triggers: a retrospective review of ED visits using an electronic medical record. Am J Emerg Med 29:1074–1082. https://doi.org/10.1016/J.AJEM.2010.06.034

33. Liu GC, Wilson JS, Qi R, Ying J (2007) Green neighborhoods, food retail and childhood overweight: differences by population density. Am J Health Promot 21:317–325. https://doi.org/10.4278/0890-1171-21.4S.317

34. Maas J, Verheij RA, De Vries S et al (2009) Morbidity is related to a green living environment. J Epidemiol Community Health 63:967–973. https://doi.org/10.1136/JECH.2008.079038

35. Casey JA, Curriero FC, Cosgrove SE et al (2013) High-density livestock operations, crop field application of manure, and risk of community-associated methicillin-resistant *Staphylococcus aureus* infection in Pennsylvania. JAMA Intern Med 173:1980–1990. https://doi.org/10.1001/JAMAINTERNMED.2013.10408

36. Casey JA, Savitz DA, Rasmussen SG et al (2016) Unconventional natural gas development and birth outcomes in Pennsylvania, USA. Epidemiology 27:163–172. https://doi.org/10.1097/EDE.0000000000000387

37. Duncan DT, Sharifi M, Melly SJ et al (2014) Characteristics of walkable built environments and BMI z scores in children: evidence from a large electronic health record database. Environ Health Perspect 122:1359–1365. https://doi.org/10.1289/ehp.1307704

38. Liu AY, Curriero FC, Glass TA et al (2013) The contextual influence of coal abandoned mine lands in communities and type 2 diabetes in Pennsylvania. Health Place 22:115–122. https://doi.org/10.1016/J.HEALTHPLACE.2013.03.012

39. Roth C, Foraker RE, Payne PRO, Embi PJ (2014) Community-level determinants of obesity: harnessing the power of electronic health records for retrospective data analysis. BMC Med Inform Decis Mak 14:36. https://doi.org/10.1186/1472-6947-14-36/TABLES/2

40. Schwartz BS, Stewart WF, Godby S et al (2011) Body mass index and the built and social environments in children and adolescents using electronic health records. Am J Prev Med 41:e17–e28. https://doi.org/10.1016/j.amepre.2011.06.038

41. Smit LAM, van der Sman-de BF, Opstal-van Winden AWJ et al (2012) Q fever and pneumonia in an area with a high livestock density: a large population-based study. PLoS One 7:e38843. https://doi.org/10.1371/JOURNAL.PONE.0038843

42. Sartorius N (2007) Stigmatized illnesses and health care. Croat Med J 48:396–397

43. Betancourt T, Scorza P, Kanyanganzi F et al (2014) HIV and child mental health: a case–control study in Rwanda. Pediatrics 134:e464–e472. https://doi.org/10.1542/peds.2013-2734

44. Biederman DJ, Modarai F, Gamble J et al (2019) Identifying patients experiencing homelessness in an electronic health record and assessing qualification for medical respite: a five-year retrospective review. J Health Care Poor Underserved 30:297–309. https://doi.org/10.1353/HPU.2019.0022

45. Blewett DR, Barnett GO, Chueh HC (1999) Experience with an electronic health record for a homeless population. Proc AMIA Symp 1999:481–485

46. Stella SA, Hanratty R, Davidson AJ et al (2024) Improving identification of patients experiencing homelessness in the electronic health record: a curated registry approach. J Gen Intern Med 39:3113. https://doi.org/10.1007/S11606-024-08909-1

47. Birkhead GS, Klompas M, Shah NR (2015) Uses of electronic health records for public health surveillance to advance public health. Annu Rev Public Health 36:345–359. https://doi.org/10.1146/ANNUREV-PUBLHEALTH-031914-122747

48. Schwalbe N, Wahl B, Song J, Lehtimaki S (2020) Data sharing and global public health: defining what we mean by data. Front Digit Health 2:612339. https://doi.org/10.3389/FDGTH.2020.612339/BIBTEX

49. Callahan A, Fries JA, Ré C et al (2019) Medical device surveillance with electronic health records. NPJ Digit Med 2:94. https://doi.org/10.1038/S41746-019-0168-Z

50. Ponjoan A, Garre-Olmo J, Blanch J et al (2019) Epidemiology of dementia: prevalence and incidence estimates using validated electronic health records from primary care. Clin Epidemiol 11:217–228. https://doi.org/10.2147/CLEP.S186590

51. Cocoros NM, Fuller CC, Adimadhyam S et al (2021) A COVID-19-ready public health surveillance system: the Food and Drug Administration's sentinel system. Pharmacoepidemiol Drug Saf 30:827–837. https://doi.org/10.1002/PDS.5240

52. Flood TL, Zhao YQ, Tomayko EJ et al (2015) Electronic health records and community health surveillance of childhood obesity. Am J Prev Med 48:234–240. https://doi.org/10.1016/J.AMEPRE.2014.10.020

53. Moore TJ, Furberg CD (2015) Electronic health data for postmarket surveillance: a vision not realized. Drug Saf 38:601–610. https://doi.org/10.1007/S40264-015-0305-9

54. Bentley SD, Lo SW (2021) Global genomic pathogen surveillance to inform vaccine strategies: a decade-long expedition in pneumococcal genomics. Genome Med 13:84. https://doi.org/10.1186/S13073-021-00901-2

55. GPS (2022) GPS: global pneumococcal sequencing project. https://www.pneumogen.net/gps/project_outline.html. Accessed 10 Dec 2023

56. Deng X, Den Bakker HC, Hendriksen RS (2016) Genomic epidemiology: whole-genome-sequencing-powered surveillance and outbreak investigation of foodborne bacterial pathogens. Annu Rev Food Sci Technol 7:353–374. https://doi.org/10.1146/ANNUREV-FOOD-041715-033259

57. Centers for Disease Control and Prevention (CDC) (2021) About PulseNet. https://www.cdc.gov/pulsenet/about/index.html. Accessed 10 Dec 2023
58. Centers for Disease Control and Prevention (CDC) (2016) PulseNet International. https://www.cdc.gov/pulsenet/participants/international/index.html. Accessed 10 Dec 2023
59. Centers for Disease Control and Prevention (CDC) (2017) PulseNet International: on the path to implementing whole-genome sequencing for foodborne disease surveillance. https://www.cdc.gov/pulsenet/pdf/pulsenet-international-wgs.pdf. Accessed 10 Dec 2023
60. Stieb DM, Boot CR, Turner MC (2017) Promise and pitfalls in the application of big data to occupational and environmental health. BMC Public Health 17:372. https://doi.org/10.1186/S12889-017-4286-8
61. Dini G, Bragazzi NL, Montecucco A et al (2019) Big data in occupational medicine: the convergence of -omics sciences, participatory research and e-health. Med Lav 110:102–114. https://doi.org/10.23749/MDL.V110I2.7765
62. European Centre for Disease Prevention and Control (ECDC) (2021) EpiPulse - the European surveillance portal for infectious diseases. https://www.ecdc.europa.eu/en/publications-data/epipulse-european-surveillance-portal-infectious-diseases. Accessed 10 Dec 2023
63. Montalti M, Kawalec A, Leoni E, Dallolio L (2020) Measles immunization policies and vaccination coverage in EU/EEA countries over the last decade. Vaccines (Basel) 8:86. https://doi.org/10.3390/VACCINES8010086
64. Donken R, Bogaards JA, van der Klis FRM et al (2016) An exploration of individual- and population-level impact of the 2-dose HPV vaccination schedule in preadolescent girls. Hum Vaccin Immunother 12:1381–1393. https://doi.org/10.1080/21645515.2016.1160978
65. Ravensbergen SJ, Nellums LB, Hargreaves S et al (2019) National approaches to the vaccination of recently arrived migrants in Europe: a comparative policy analysis across 32 European countries. Travel Med Infect Dis 27:33–38. https://doi.org/10.1016/J.TMAID.2018.10.011
66. European Centre for Disease Prevention and Control (ECDC) (2023) Antimicrobial consumption dashboard (ESAC-Net). https://www.ecdc.europa.eu/en/antimicrobial-consumption/surveillance-and-disease-data/database. Accessed 10 Dec 2023
67. Robertson J, Vlahović-Palčevski V, Iwamoto K et al (2021) Variations in the consumption of antimicrobial medicines in the European region, 2014-2018: findings and implications from ESAC-net and WHO Europe. Front Pharmacol 12:639207. https://doi.org/10.3389/FPHAR.2021.639207
68. Adriaenssens N, Bruyndonckx R, Versporten A et al (2021) Consumption of quinolones in the community, European Union/European Economic Area, 1997-2017. J Antimicrob Chemother 76:II37–II44. https://doi.org/10.1093/JAC/DKAB176
69. European Centre for Disease Prevention and Control (ECDC) (2017) The European Surveillance System (TESSy). https://www.ecdc.europa.eu/en/publications-data/european-surveillance-system-tessy. Accessed 10 Dec 2023
70. European Centre for Disease Prevention and Control (ECDC) (2023) Surveillance Atlas of infectious diseases. https://www.ecdc.europa.eu/en/surveillance-atlas-infectious-diseases. Accessed 10 Dec 2023
71. Whittaker R, Dias JG, Ramliden M et al (2017) The epidemiology of invasive meningococcal disease in EU/EEA countries, 2004-2014. Vaccine 35:2034–2041. https://doi.org/10.1016/J.VACCINE.2017.03.007
72. Lake IR, Colón-González FJ, Takkinen J et al (2019) Exploring Campylobacter seasonality across Europe using The European Surveillance System (TESSy), 2008 to 2016. Euro Surveill 24:1800028. https://doi.org/10.2807/1560-7917.ES.2019.24.13.180028
73. Snacken R, Brown C (2015) New developments of influenza surveillance in Europe. Euro Surveill 20:21020. https://doi.org/10.2807/ESE.20.04.21020-EN
74. European Medicine Agency (EMA) About us. https://www.ema.europa.eu/en/about-us. Accessed 26 Sep 2024

75. European Medicines Agency (2001) EudraVigilance. https://www.ema.europa.eu/en/human-regulatory-overview/research-and-development/pharmacovigilance-research-and-development/eudravigilance. Accessed 10 Dec 2023

76. Postigo R, Brosch S, Slattery J et al (2018) EudraVigilance medicines safety database: publicly accessible data for research and public health protection. Drug Saf 41:665–675. https://doi.org/10.1007/S40264-018-0647-1/TABLES/3

77. Abbattista M, Martinelli I, Peyvandi F (2021) Comparison of adverse drug reactions among four COVID-19 vaccines in Europe using the EudraVigilance database: thrombosis at unusual sites. J Thromb Haemost 19:2554–2558. https://doi.org/10.1111/JTH.15493

78. Tobaiqy M, Maclure K, Elkout H, Stewart D (2021) Thrombotic adverse events reported for Moderna, Pfizer and Oxford-AstraZeneca COVID-19 vaccines: comparison of occurrence and clinical outcomes in the EudraVigilance Database. Vaccines 9:1326. https://doi.org/10.3390/VACCINES9111326

79. Isai A, Durand J, Le Meur S et al (2012) Autoimmune disorders after immunization with Influenza A/H1N1 vaccines with and without adjuvant: EudraVigilance data and literature review. Vaccine 30:7123–7129. https://doi.org/10.1016/J.VACCINE.2012.09.032

80. Liang D, Sessa M (2022) Postmarketing safety surveillance of erenumab: new insight from Eudravigilance. Expert Opin Drug Saf 21:1205–1210. https://doi.org/10.1080/14740338.2022.2049231

81. Chiappini S, Vickers-Smith R, Guirguis A et al (2022) Pharmacovigilance signals of the opioid epidemic over 10 years: data mining methods in the analysis of pharmacovigilance datasets collecting adverse drug reactions (ADRs) reported to EudraVigilance (EV) and the FDA Adverse Event Reporting System (FAERS). Pharmaceuticals 15:675. https://doi.org/10.3390/PH15060675/S1

82. Delsaux P (2022) Preparing Europe for future health threats and crises – the European Health Emergency and Preparedness Authority; improving EU preparedness and response in the area of medical countermeasures. Euro Surveill 27:2200893. https://doi.org/10.2807/1560-7917.ES.2022.27.47.2200893

83. European Commission (2022) HEALTH UNION: identifying top 3 priority health threats. https://health.ec.europa.eu/system/files/2022-07/hera_factsheet_health-threat_mcm.pdf. Accessed 21 Dec 2023

84. Centers for Disease Control and Prevention (CDC) (2022) About CDC. https://www.cdc.gov/about/. Accessed 11 Dec 2023

85. Centers for Disease Control and Prevention (CDC) (2023) BEAM (Bacteria, Enterics, Amoeba, and Mycotics) Dashboard. https://www.cdc.gov/ncezid/dfwed/BEAM-dashboard.html. Accessed 11 Dec 2023

86. Centers for Disease Control and Prevention (CDC) (2023) Disability and Health Data System (DHDS). https://www.cdc.gov/ncbddd/disabilityandhealth/dhds/index.html. Accessed 11 Dec 2023

87. Centers for Disease Control and Prevention (CDC) (2023) COVID-19 Case Surveillance Public Use Data with Geography | Data | Centers for Disease Control and Prevention. https://data.cdc.gov/Case-Surveillance/COVID-19-Case-Surveillance-Public-Use-Data-with-Ge/n8mc-b4w4/about_data. Accessed 11 Dec 2023

88. Gostin LO (2023) The World Health Organization on its 75th anniversary. JAMA Health Forum 4:E231568. https://doi.org/10.1001/JAMAHEALTHFORUM.2023.1568

89. World Health Organization (WHO) (2023) Who we are. https://www.who.int/about/who-we-are. Accessed 11 Dec 2023

90. World Health Organization (WHO) (2023) Leading causes of death and disability 2000-2019: a visual summary. https://www.who.int/data/stories/leading-causes-of-death-and-disability-2000-2019-a-visual-summary. Accessed 11 Dec 2023

91. World Health Organization (WHO) (2023) Global health estimates: life expectancy and leading causes of death and disability. https://www.who.int/data/gho/data/themes/mortality-and-global-health-estimates. Accessed 11 Dec 2023

92. World Health Organization (WHO) (2023) World Health Statistics. https://www.who.int/data/gho/publications/world-health-statistics. Accessed 11 Dec 2023

93. World Health Organization (WHO) (2023) WHO Mortality Database (MDB). https://platform.who.int/mortality. Accessed 11 Dec 2023

94. Peto R, Boreham J, Lopez AD et al (1992) Mortality from tobacco in developed countries: indirect estimation from national vital statistics. Lancet 339:1268–1278. https://doi.org/10.1016/0140-6736(92)91600-D

95. World Health Organization (WHO) (2023) About the outbreak toolkit project. https://www.who.int/emergencies/outbreak-toolkit/about. Accessed 11 Dec 2023

96. World Health Organization (WHO) (2023) Global influenza programme. https://www.who.int/tools/flunet. Accessed 11 Dec 2023

97. OECD (2024). How we work. https://www.oecd.org/en/about/how-we-work.html. Accessed 31 Jan 2025

98. OECD (2024). Health. https://www.oecd.org/en/topics/health.html. Accessed 31 Jan 2025

99. OECD (2023) Ready for the next crisis? Investing in health system resilience. OECD Health Policy Studies, OECD, Paris

100. OECD iLibrary (2023) OECD Health Statistics. https://www.oecd-ilibrary.org/social-issues-migration-health/data/oecd-health-statistics_health-data-en. Accessed 11 Dec 2023

101. OECD (2021) Healthcare quality and outcomes indicators. https://www.oecd.org/health/health-care-quality-outcomes-indicators.htm. Accessed 11 Dec 2023

102. NSW Government (2021) HealthStats NSW. https://www.healthstats.nsw.gov.au/#/home. Accessed 11 Dec 2023

103. Garbi M (2021) National Institute for Health and Care Excellence clinical guidelines development principles and processes. Heart 107:949–953. https://doi.org/10.1136/HEARTJNL-2020-318661

104. National Institute for Health and Care Excellence (NICE) (2023) Published guidance, NICE advice and quality standards. https://www.nice.org.uk/guidance/published?ngt=Cancer%20service%20guidelines&ngt=Clinical%20guidelines&ngt=Medicines%20practice%20guidelines&ngt=Public%20health%20guidelines&ngt=Safe%20staffing%20guidelines&ngt=Social%20care%20guidelines&ndt=Guidance. Accessed 11 Dec 2023

105. Australian Government AI of H and W (AIHW) (2023) About us - Australian Institute of Health and Welfare. https://www.aihw.gov.au/about-us. Accessed 11 Dec 2023

106. Smith M, Saunders R, Stuckhardt L, McGinnis J (2013) Best care at lower cost: the path to continuously learning health care in America. National Academies Press, Washington, DC. https://doi.org/10.17226/13444

107. Budrionis A, Bellika JG (2016) The learning healthcare system: where are we now? A systematic review. J Biomed Inform 64:87–92. https://doi.org/10.1016/J.JBI.2016.09.018

108. Enticott J, Johnson A, Teede H (2021) Learning health systems using data to drive healthcare improvement and impact: a systematic review. BMC Health Serv Res 21:200. https://doi.org/10.1186/S12913-021-06215-8

109. OECD (2017) New health technologies: managing access, value and sustainability. OECD, Paris

110. Eichler HG, Bloechl-Daum B, Broich K et al (2019) Data rich, information poor: can we use electronic health records to create a learning healthcare system for pharmaceuticals? Clin Pharmacol Ther 105:912–922. https://doi.org/10.1002/CPT.1226

111. Hu J, Perer A, Wang F (2016) Data driven analytics for personalized healthcare. In: Weaver C, Ball M, Kim G, Kiel J (eds) Healthcare information management systems. Health Informatics. Springer, Cham, pp 529–554

112. Perer A, Gotz D (2013) Data-driven exploration of care plans for patients. https://doi.org/10.1145/2468356.2468434

113. Ginsburg GS, McCarthy JJ (2001) Personalized medicine: revolutionizing drug discovery and patient care. Trends Biotechnol 19:491–496. https://doi.org/10.1016/S0167-7799(01)01814-5

114. Jain KK (2002) Personalized medicine. Curr Opin Mol Ther 4:548–558. https://doi. org/10.1177/0022034512449171
115. Abul-Husn NS, Kenny EE (2019) Personalized medicine and the power of electronic health records. Cell 177:58–69. https://doi.org/10.1016/J.CELL.2019.02.039
116. National Human Genome Research Institute (2012) International HapMap Project. https:// www.genome.gov/10001688/internationalhopmap-project. Accessed 11 Dec 2023
117. Alfian G, Syafrudin M, Ijaz MF et al (2018) A personalized healthcare monitoring system for diabetic patients by utilizing BLE-based sensors and real-time data processing. Sensors (Basel) 18. https://doi.org/10.3390/S18072183
118. Lv N, Xiao L, Simmons ML et al (2017) Personalized hypertension management using patient-generated health data integrated with electronic health records (EMPOWER-H): six-month pre-post study. J Med Internet Res 19:e311. https://doi.org/10.2196/JMIR.7831
119. Lee J, Maslove DM, Dubin JA (2015) Personalized mortality prediction driven by electronic medical data and a patient similarity metric. PLoS One 10:e0127428. https://doi.org/10.1371/JOURNAL.PONE.0127428
120. Relling MV, Evans WE (2015) Pharmacogenomics in the clinic. Nature 526:343–350. https://doi.org/10.1038/NATURE15817
121. Atasoy H, Greenwood BN, McCullough JS (2019) The digitization of patient care: a review of the effects of electronic health records on health care quality and utilization. Annu Rev Public Health 40:487–500. https://doi.org/10.1146/ANNUREV-PUBL HEALTH-040218-044206
122. Romano MJ, Stafford RS (2011) Electronic health records and clinical decision support systems: impact on national ambulatory care quality. Arch Intern Med 171:897–903. https://doi. org/10.1001/ARCHINTERNMED.2010.527
123. Li E, Clarke J, Ashrafian H et al (2022) The impact of electronic health record interoperability on safety and quality of care in high-income countries: systematic review. J Med Internet Res 24:e38144. https://doi.org/10.2196/38144
124. McDonald KM, Davies SM, Haberland CA et al (2008) Preliminary assessment of pediatric health care quality and patient safety in the United States using readily available administrative data. Pediatrics 122:e416–e425. https://doi.org/10.1542/PEDS.2007-2477
125. Weill Cornell Medicine, Department of Anesthesiology (2016) Quality and patient safety. https://anesthesiology.weill.cornell.edu/about-us/quality-and-patient-safety. Accessed 11 Dec 2023
126. Mukasa CDM, Kovacheva VP (2022) Development and implementation of databases to track patient and safety outcomes. Curr Opin Anaesthesiol 35:710–716. https://doi.org/10.1097/ACO.0000000000001201
127. Gupta PM (2023) The role of big data in smart healthcare. Int J Internet Things 11:11–18
128. Kim E, Rubinstein SM, Nead KT et al (2019) The evolving use of electronic health records (EHR) for research. Semin Radiat Oncol 29:354–361. https://doi.org/10.1016/J. SEMRADONC.2019.05.010
129. Stewart R, Soremekun M, Perera G et al (2009) The South London and Maudsley NHS Foundation Trust Biomedical Research Centre (SLAM BRC) case register: development and descriptive data. BMC Psychiatry 9:51. https://doi.org/10.1186/1471-244X-9-51
130. Perera G, Broadbent M, Callard F et al (2016) Cohort profile of the South London and Maudsley NHS Foundation Trust Biomedical Research Centre (SLaM BRC) Case Register: current status and recent enhancement of an Electronic Mental Health Record-derived data resource. BMJ Open 6:e008721. https://doi.org/10.1136/BMJOPEN-2015-008721
131. Tulloch AD, Fearon P, David AS (2011) Residential mobility among patients admitted to acute psychiatric wards. Health Place 17:859–866. https://doi.org/10.1016/J. HEALTHPLACE.2011.05.006
132. Tulloch AD, Fearon P, David AS (2012) Timing, prevalence, determinants and outcomes of homelessness among patients admitted to acute psychiatric wards. Soc Psychiatry Psychiatr Epidemiol 47:1181–1191. https://doi.org/10.1007/S00127-011-0414-4

133. Fusar-Poli P, Díaz-Caneja CM, Patel R et al (2016) Services for people at high risk improve outcomes in patients with first episode psychosis. Acta Psychiatr Scand 133:76–85. https:// doi.org/10.1111/ACPS.12480

134. Patel R, Shetty H, Jackson R et al (2015) Delays before diagnosis and initiation of treatment in patients presenting to mental health services with bipolar disorder. PLoS One 10:e0126530. https://doi.org/10.1371/JOURNAL.PONE.0126530

135. Lin WC, Chen JS, Chiang MF, Hribar MR (2020) Applications of artificial intelligence to electronic health record data in ophthalmology. Transl Vis Sci Technol 9:13. https://doi. org/10.1167/TVST.9.2.13

136. Davis KAS, Sudlow CLM, Hotopf M (2016) Can mental health diagnoses in administrative data be used for research? A systematic review of the accuracy of routinely collected diagnoses. BMC Psychiatry 16:263. https://doi.org/10.1186/S12888-016-0963-X

137. Xu H, Aldrich MC, Chen Q et al (2015) Validating drug repurposing signals using electronic health records: a case study of metformin associated with reduced cancer mortality. J Am Med Inform Assoc 22:179–191. https://doi.org/10.1136/AMIAJNL-2014-002649

138. Gordon DE, Hiatt J, Bouhaddou M et al (2020) Comparative host-coronavirus protein interaction networks reveal panviral disease mechanisms. Science 370:eabe9403. https://doi. org/10.1126/science.abe9403

139. Kim H, Xu H, George E et al (2020) Combining PARP with ATR inhibition overcomes PARP inhibitor and platinum resistance in ovarian cancer models. Nat Commun 11:3726. https:// doi.org/10.1038/S41467-020-17127-2

140. Zhu Y, Xu Y, Helseth DL et al (2015) Zodiac: a comprehensive depiction of genetic interactions in cancer by integrating TCGA data. J Natl Cancer Inst 107:djv129. https://doi. org/10.1093/JNCI/DJV129

141. Yao L, Zhang Y, Li Y et al (2011) Electronic health records: implications for drug discovery. Drug Discov Today 16:594–599. https://doi.org/10.1016/J.DRUDIS.2011.05.009

142. Hanauer DA, Rhodes DR, Chinnaiyan AM (2009) Exploring clinical associations using "-omics" based enrichment analyses. PLoS One 4:e5203. https://doi.org/10.1371/JOURNAL. PONE.0005203

143. Jonas WB, Rapoza CP, Blair WF (1996) The effect of niacinamide on osteoarthritis: a pilot study. Inflamm Res 45:330–334. https://doi.org/10.1007/BF02252945

144. Ma A, Medenica M (1983) Response of generalized granuloma annulare to high-dose niacinamide. Arch Dermatol 119:836–839

145. The Center for Open Data Enterprise (2019) Sharing and utilizing health data for AI applications. https://healthdatasharing.org/wp-content/uploads/2020/07/RT1-AI-Summary-Report-FINAL-2020.07.28.pdf. Accessed 11 Dec 2023

146. Teltsch DY, Fazeli Farsani S, Swain RS et al (2019) Development and validation of algorithms to identify newly diagnosed type 1 and type 2 diabetes in pediatric population using electronic medical records and claims data. Pharmacoepidemiol Drug Saf 28:234–243. https://doi.org/10.1002/PDS.4728

147. Kharbanda EO, Vazquez-Benitez G, DeSilva MB et al (2021) Developing algorithms for identifying major structural birth defects using automated electronic health data. Pharmacoepidemiol Drug Saf 30:266–274. https://doi.org/10.1002/PDS.5177

148. Yuan Q, Cai T, Hong C et al (2021) Performance of a machine learning algorithm using electronic health record data to identify and estimate survival in a longitudinal cohort of patients with lung cancer. JAMA Netw Open 4:e2114723. https://doi.org/10.1001/ JAMANETWORKOPEN.2021.14723

149. Lin E, Balogh R, Cobigo V et al (2013) Using administrative health data to identify individuals with intellectual and developmental disabilities: a comparison of algorithms. J Intellect Disabil Res 57:462–477. https://doi.org/10.1111/JIR.12002

150. Ravaut M, Harish V, Sadeghi H et al (2021) Development and validation of a machine learning model using administrative health data to predict onset of type 2 diabetes. JAMA Netw Open 4:e2111315. https://doi.org/10.1001/JAMANETWORKOPEN.2021.11315

151. Gianfrancesco MA, Tamang S, Yazdany J, Schmajuk G (2018) Potential biases in machine learning algorithms using electronic health record data. JAMA Intern Med 178:1544–1547. https://doi.org/10.1001/JAMAINTERNMED.2018.3763

152. Adams KF, Johnson EA, Chubak J et al (2015) Development of an algorithm to classify colonoscopy indication from coded health care data. EGEMS (Wash DC) 3:1171. https://doi.org/10.13063/2327-9214.1171

153. Gharehchopogh FS, Peyman M, Parvin H (2012) Application of decision tree algorithm for data mining in healthcare operations: a case study. Int J Comput Appl 52:21–26

154. Oh J, Yun K, Maoz U et al (2019) Identifying depression in the National Health and Nutrition Examination Survey data using a deep learning algorithm. J Affect Disord 257:623–631. https://doi.org/10.1016/J.JAD.2019.06.034

155. Philip G, Djerboua M, Carlone D, Flemming JA (2020) Validation of a hierarchical algorithm to define chronic liver disease and cirrhosis etiology in administrative healthcare data. PLoS One 15:e0229218. https://doi.org/10.1371/JOURNAL.PONE.0229218

156. Benchimol EI, Guttmann A, Mack DR et al (2014) Validation of international algorithms to identify adults with inflammatory bowel disease in health administrative data from Ontario, Canada. J Clin Epidemiol 67:887–896. https://doi.org/10.1016/J.JCLINEPI.2014.02.019

157. Farran B, Channanath AM, Behbehani K, Thanaraj TA (2013) Predictive models to assess risk of type 2 diabetes, hypertension and comorbidity: machine-learning algorithms and validation using national health data from Kuwait--a cohort study. BMJ Open 3:e002457. https://doi.org/10.1136/BMJOPEN-2012-002457

158. Farran B, AlWotayan R, Alkandari H et al (2019) Use of noninvasive parameters and machine-learning algorithms for predicting future risk of type 2 diabetes: a retrospective cohort study of health data from Kuwait. Front Endocrinol (Lausanne) 10:624. https://doi.org/10.3389/FENDO.2019.00624

159. Mohamadlou H, Lynn-Palevsky A, Barton C et al (2018) Prediction of acute kidney injury with a machine learning algorithm using electronic health record data. Can J Kidney Health Dis 5:2054358118776326. https://doi.org/10.1177/2054358118776326

160. Zhang B, Ren J, Cheng Y et al (2019) Health data driven on continuous blood pressure prediction based on gradient boosting decision tree algorithm. IEEE Access 7:32423–32433. https://doi.org/10.1109/ACCESS.2019.2902217

161. Miotto R et al (2016) Deep patient: an unsupervised representation to predict the future of patients from the electronic health records. Sci Rep 6:26094. https://doi.org/10.1038/srep26094

162. Tsui FR, Shi L, Ruiz V, Ryan ND, Biernesser C, Iyengar S, Walsh CG, Brent DA (2021) Natural language processing and machine learning of electronic health records for prediction of first-time suicide attempts. JAMIA Open 4(1):ooab011. https://doi.org/10.1093/jamiaopen/ooab011

163. Carson NJ, Mullin B, Sanchez MJ, Lu F, Yang K, Menezes M, Cook BL (2019) Identification of suicidal behavior among psychiatrically hospitalized adolescents using natural language processing and machine learning of electronic health records. PLoS One 14(2):e0211116. https://doi.org/10.1371/journal.pone.0211116

164. Feller DJ, Zucker J, Yin MT, Gordon P, Elhadad N (2018) Using clinical notes and natural language processing for automated HIV risk assessment. J Acquir Immune Defic Syndr 77(2):160. https://www.ncbi.nlm.nih.gov/pmc/articles/PMC5762388/

165. Deng Y, Pacheco JA, Chung A et al (2021) Natural language processing to identify lupus nephritis phenotype in electronic health records. BMC Med Inform Decis Mak 10.48550/arXiv.2112.10821

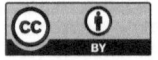

Chapter 3
Enabling Factors and Opportunities to Maximize Health Data Reuse

3.1 Goal of Digital Maturity for Healthcare System Advancement

The potential for improved efficiency in current healthcare systems is related to an increased need for metrics and indicators to monitor and control the implementation of digital health. However, the identification and application of metrics related to the governance, availability, and reuse of electronic health data have emerged as common challenges, not only at the micro level but also at the macro- or country level. Healthcare providers' inability to communicate with each other electronically and exchange health data is notable for many national health systems around the world. For example, in Europe, addressing these issues will project a pathway of improved European health service provision with a shift in healthcare processes and activities for most countries [1]. However, some of the goals can be reached with the implementation of a mature digitally based data-driven approach. These include (1) the increase in indicators available to compare the performance of multiple different institutions or health systems at different levels (regional, national, or international), (2) the development of telehealth technologies that allow the treatment of multiple populations at the same time or with a higher patient/provider ratio, and (3) the development of metrics that assess health disparities, etc. [1]. In the context of digital health implementation at the country level, digital maturity, which is the implementation of large-scale digital health programmes [2], serves as a building block for multiple potential applications of digital health. The concept of "digital health maturity" offers a framework for coordinating digital efforts towards a variety of objectives, such as increasing patient satisfaction, eradicating health disparities, directing resource allocation and cost containment, and improving working conditions for healthcare professionals. Countries can align their knowledge, abilities, and resources to systematically develop, implement, and assess standard-based, interoperable digital health systems and programmes to support and sustain their health priorities by assessing their level of digital health maturity. New frameworks

© The Author(s) 2025
F. Cascini, *Secondary Use of Electronic Health Data*, SpringerBriefs in Public Health, https://doi.org/10.1007/978-3-031-88497-9_3

and metrics are nevertheless required to evaluate digital maturity with respect to these complex objectives. The use of digital health tools to improve health systems across the board must be acknowledged as a potential source of data for measuring and tracking indicators of digital health maturity, such as effects on care, quality enhancement, development of health professionals, and risk management [3]. At the country level, this becomes more important as the complexity of healthcare population needs increases, therefore requiring the rearrangement of processes to adapt properly to the new healthcare provision framework that has taken place individually in each region and country. The level of preparation of each system for these rearrangement processes can be seen as a broad level of definition of digital maturity.

Healthcare services differ from other conventional industrial services in terms of population impact, dynamics, interdisciplinarity, and process control (human-centred). Therefore, in the healthcare sector, digital maturity requires not only adopting general models for digital maturity but also using domain-specific models for this sector [4]. This need has been recognized by some authors, who have supported the development and evaluation of maturity models for healthcare, including models specifically developed for locally operating public health agencies, once digitalization appeared to be a critical task enabling coordinated crisis responses to health-related threats [5]. Some countries, such as the UK, support the concept of digital maturity not only for the primary use of data (which certainly play a key role in the future of healthcare systems) but also, more importantly, in the field of secondary use of health data to support governance and maximize the proper use of health information at the country level [6]. This is the case for the UK National Health Service (NHS), which has devoted efforts for more than 5 years to adapting the national health system to increase digitalization while preserving data privacy and security in secondary use cases and allowing, among other things, patients to manage their own data with opt-out strategies as well as improving data access for public interest purposes. The overall goal is to improve outcomes and provide informed responsive care [7]. Countries that have not implemented digital transformation of healthcare at full capacity should work with a roadmap or informed pathway to meaningfully change the current capabilities of their digital landscape, aiming for a complete digital change in the health sector as a whole [8].

Digital maturity enables countries to systematically design, execute, and assess interoperable, standard-based digital health programmes to maintain and support their foremost health priorities [1, 9]. There is a factual relationship between digital maturity and the positive impact on healthcare improvement and effectiveness [10, 11]. This relationship has been highlighted by recognized organizations such as the American Hospital Association, which has emphasized data-driven models for the creation of a new care delivery model needed today and has designed a maturity framework on the basis of three different capabilities: (1) the status of data assets, (2) data storage, and (3) data analytics and infrastructure [12]. Other reports have also emphasized the current healthcare marketplace that is in need of data-driven innovation, which will require digital maturity levels at a minimum for this to take place. In fact, it is predicted that there will be a worldwide shortfall of 18 million health workers by 2030, which calls for acceleration in the adoption of digital technologies, with new concepts such as nanobots performing medical interventions for >50 patients at the same time while being supervised by a medical engineer hundreds of miles away [13]. Although widely acknowledged, these trends will require the implementation of new transformation tools (some of which already exist) that will improve access to and efficiency of care while reducing costs at the same time. Both existing and future digital technologies have a common characteristic: the need for a sufficient level of digital maturity in the country and/or organizations to implement technological innovation and support digital tool utilization. In some cases, this becomes more important, requiring an expert level for all three capabilities enlisted by the American Hospital Association. Digital maturity is therefore seen as necessary at both the individual and systematic levels to ensure successful, scalable, and sustainable digital transformation in healthcare. This is a continuous and already evolving process. In fact, at the present time, we are already seeing part of this transformation in healthcare. Digital technologies are leading the transformation of the healthcare sector and are generating new models of health service delivery ranging from prevention to personalized medicine and precision healthcare [14].

3.2   Opportunity of Artificial Intelligence for Public Health Purposes[1]

The digitalization of healthcare systems and the implementation of health data-driven approaches allow the development of novel, targeted public health solutions. The growing amount of health data generated every year makes big data platforms essential tools for data management and analytics. Although various artificial intelligence (AI) systems are being developed with the aid of such platforms, they generally share similar objectives, such as assisting health systems in response to specific emerging health demands; designing healthcare services that are able to scale their provision according to the growth of populations; improving public health resilience and responsiveness to promptly control epidemic-related emergencies; and better differentiating patient communities through risk stratification and informing individual decision-making, both of which are essential for the personalized medicine movement. The development of AI and its promising applications allows targeted public health interventions such as screening and prevention activities, which are based on specific population subgroups' needs to maximize their effectiveness and relevance.

---

[1] Most of this section has published previously in: Cascini, F., Buttigieg, S., Pastorino, R., Ricciardi, W., Boccia, S. (2023). Personalized Medicine Through Artificial Intelligence: A Public Health Perspective. In: Cesario, A., D'Oria, M., Auffray, C., Scambia, G. (eds) *Personalized Medicine Meets Artificial Intelligence*. Springer, Cham. https://doi.org/10.1007/978-3-031-32614-1_1. Reproduced with permission of Springer Nature.

Consistent progress has also been made in various health-related fields, from drug discovery to medical imaging, assisting healthcare professionals and providers in reducing medical errors, and allowing clinicians to focus on solving complex cases. For example, AI development for health is creating terrific support to improve the early diagnosis of various diseases. This is particularly explored in the field of oncology, where AI is being evaluated for use in radiological diagnoses, such as in whole-body imaging, colonoscopies, and mammograms. AI can also aid in optimizing radiological treatment dosing, recognizing malignant disease in dermatology or clinical pathology, and guiding RNA and DNA sequencing for immunotherapy [15]. In general, AI developments in early diagnosis are being studied in most health-related fields, such as in the early diagnosis of diabetic retinopathy, cardiovascular disease, liver disease, and neurological disorders [16]. Currently, there are only a handful of prospective clinical trials on the effectiveness of AI in early diagnosis, with some showing promise of equivalent detection ability to that of human professionals in specific tasks, with even fewer focusing on the potential benefits of human–machine partnerships. One of the risks in relying excessively on AI and machine learning algorithms is the development of an automation bias, where medical practitioners might not consider other important aspects in patient care and overlook errors that should have been spotted by human-guided decision-making [17].

AI can also be used to digitalize and store traditional paper medical records and process large amounts of data from images and other types of inputs or signals (such as motion data or sound data). Steps in image and signal processing algorithms typically include signal feature analysis and data classification via tools such as artificial neural networks, which work via complex layers of decision nodes [18]. Medical imaging is one of the most rapidly developing areas of AI application in healthcare. While improving automated image interpretation and analysis are a priority, other important aspects of AI application to medical imaging are being explored, such as data security and user privacy solutions for medical image analysis, deep learning algorithms for the restoration or reconstruction, and segmentation of complex images and the creation of fuzzy sets or rough sets in medical image analysis [19, 20]. With health systems becoming increasingly complex, the administration and management of care are becoming increasingly laborious. AI can be used to assist personnel in complex logistical tasks, such as optimization of the medical supply chain, to assume mundane, repetitive tasks or to support complex decision-making [21]. This is made possible by a combination of AI advancements in the fields of natural language processing, automated scheduling and planning, and expert systems [22].

Many AI tools can be further used in specific public health programmes or in wide public health approaches to improve population well-being. For example, AI can be used for health promotion or to identify target populations or locations with "high-risk" behaviour concerning communicable and noncommunicable diseases. AI can improve the effectiveness of communication and messaging specifically directed at certain subpopulations, both in terms of its ability to recognize priority groups and its adaptiveness in creating tailor-suited messages to benefit population health (microtargeting) [23]. One example of such an application is microtargeting individuals or communities with technological, linguistic, or cultural barriers to better communicate the importance and safety of vaccinations, such as the COVID-19 vaccination [24]. AI tools could therefore be adapted to improve access to and equity of care, furthering the development of truly personalized medicine. AI can also play a leading role in performing analyses of patterns of data for health surveillance and disease detection [25–28]: AI tools can be used to identify bacterial contamination in water treatment plants, identify foodborne illnesses in restaurants or hospitals, simplify detection, and lower costs. Sensors can also be used to improve environmental health, such as by analysing air pollution patterns or using machine learning to make inferences between the physical environment and healthy behaviour [29]. Another application of AI in public health surveillance is evidence collection and its use to create mathematical models to make decisions. Although many public health institutions are not yet making full use of all possible sources of data, some fields, such as real-time health surveillance, are steadily improving. This has improved the public health outlook on pandemic preparedness and response, although the long-term ramification of such important changes will only be evident in the future [22].

The development of public health policy also proves to be fertile ground for AI, where attempts at analysing argumentation on food quality in a public health policy were attempted. This action resulted in the creation of models that output new recommendations on the basis of stakeholders' arguments by targeting specific audiences [30]. Healthcare has always depended in part on predictions, prognoses, and the use of predictive analytics. AI is just one of the more recent tools for this purpose, and many possible benefits of prediction-based healthcare rely on the use of this technology. For example, AI can be used to assess an individual's risk of disease, which could be used for the prevention of diseases and major health events. Various studies suggest that AI may improve several pathologies, such as heart failure, by utilizing predictive models and telemonitoring systems for clinical support and patient empowerment. For example, given the expected increase in the number of heart failure patients in the future due to the ageing of the population, predicting the risk of a patient having heart failure could prevent hospitalizations and readmissions, improving both patient care and hospital management, which would have a high impact on costs and time [31].

Machine learning is increasingly being applied to make predictions related to population health: the use of novel big data resources, which are ripe with different data types, may allow for improvements in the prediction algorithms necessary to navigate complex health data ecosystems successfully [32, 33]. A good example of this is the integration of data types to better understand complex associations between genetics, the environment, and disease. The Harvard group has used large administrative datasets to untangle the relationship between genetics and the environment in all diseases recorded in health insurance claims data [32]. Using biobanks and their massive datasets allows scientists around the world to discover new genetic variants (e.g. through genome-wide association studies) and novel risk factors associated with disease more efficiently and with higher sensitivity and specificity than traditional "one-at-a-time" methods do [34]. Using electronic medical record data, machine- and deep-learning algorithms have been able to predict many important clinical parameters, including suicide, Alzheimer's disease, dementia, severe sepsis, septic shock, hospital readmission, all-cause mortality, in-hospital mortality, unplanned readmission, prolonged length of stay, and final discharge diagnosis [35].

Overall, predictive models have been used much more widely by clinicians than by public health professionals. However, on closer inspection, any application that improves patient care at any level can be considered relevant to the field of public health. The ability of clinicians and healthcare providers to make better informed decisions on patient health can be improved by context-specific algorithms, which use massive quantities of clinical, physiological, epidemiological, and genetic data. Precision medicine will further benefit from these advanced algorithms, as their accuracy, timeliness and appropriateness in clinical care improve over time, decompressing our reliance on human resources. This advancement, however, still necessitates computer-literate physicians, who are up-to-date with new generation data-driven approaches. The key to the complete incorporation of AI into clinical care will therefore be the integration of human clinical judgement with advanced clinical machine learning algorithms [33].

Importantly, in addition to all the advancements in AI science and the development of AI tools, the involvement of patients remains fundamental for the secondary use of health data, with patient engagement being an important component for the improvement of care. Evidence on this topic has shown that as a patient has more access to his/her own health data, patient activation is promoted in managing their own health, which ultimately results in lower costs and better health outcomes in general [36]. Patient activation through the use of digital tools, including secondary use of health data, has been supported by evidence showing that the burden of healthcare systems can be reduced when patients are engaged and have the ability to take more control of their health. In fact, in the UK, research has shown that patients who are more active in managing their health make less use of general practice services, emergency admitted patient care, and other healthcare services than their fewer active counterparts do [37]. Trust in the health system and healthcare providers, which increases the likelihood of data altruism being performed by patients [38], is also related to patient engagement. In fact, patients' trust and data altruism for the benefits related to secondary uses of health data are shaped by a complex interrelation of factors, including the following domains: (1) the quality of care received; (2) the impact of healthcare costs; (3) the transparency and communication displayed by providers or insurers; and (4) the extent of coordination between actors, i.e. providers and insurers [39].

3.3 Importance of Common Data Spaces: The European Approach

A single European data space is being formed as part of the European strategy for dataset vision. For both personal and nonpersonal data from various sources to act as catalysts for growth and wealth creation, this vision seeks to provide a data space that will be open to receiving data from all over the world. This aim, although highly ambitious, also has the intention to serve as a solution to overcome current legal, organizational, semantic, and technical barriers for data sharing by combining the necessary tools and infrastructures across the European region that will serve to enable secure and cross-border access to key datasets in multiple thematic areas. Moreover, data spaces aim to work as decentralized-governed and standardized structures that facilitate data sharing in a trustworthy manner. These common repositories across Europe aim to facilitate the voluntary process of sharing data between its participants, thereby transforming what could be dispersed data into one connected server of information. The aim is to provide information to promote new business opportunities for the region, support innovation processes, and support the development of rules and regulations that will enable proper data reuse, secondary use, and ultimately the development of a scenario for European economic and social development [40].

Data spaces are meant to be the foundation of a vibrant data economy and the key to establishing a sovereign, interoperable, and trustworthy data sharing ecosystem. For this purpose, and owing to the complexity of data spaces, it is important to note that the development and creation of data spaces is an endeavour that requires multiple factors to align, as there is no single or organizational approach that can be applied for the establishment of European data spaces [41]. Therefore, in the understanding of the unique characteristics and complexity of data spaces, a community-based approach that involves a broad spectrum of stakeholders and promotes the interaction between multiple organizations is necessary to provide support to the multiple areas and factors needed. In the European region, the Data Spaces Business Alliance (DSBA)[2] has been established for this purpose by the Big Data Value Association (BDVA),[3] FIWARE,[4] Gaia-X,[5] and the International Data Spaces

---

[2] The Data Spaces Business Alliance (DSBA) is a pioneering initiative that brings together industry leaders to shape a data-centric future, empowering organizations and individuals to harness the full potential of their data. Available at: https://data-spaces-business-alliance.eu/

[3] The Big Data Value Association (BDVA) is a research and innovation organization led by industry, dedicated to building an innovation ecosystem that supports the data-driven and AI-powered digital transformation of Europe's economy and society. Available at: https://bdva.eu/about/

[4] FIWARE is an open-source cloud platform with a collaborative and mature ecosystem of developers, innovation Hubs, accelerators, cities, and more than 1000 SMEs and start-ups. Available at: https://digital-strategy.ec.europa.eu/en/news/fiware-european-success-story

[5] Gaia-X provides businesses, individuals, and governments with secure, transparent, and sovereign control over their data using a decentralized cloud infrastructure. Joining Gaia-X offers access to a trusted ecosystem and a collaborative community that drives innovation and scalability across industries, all while adhering to European and local regulatory standards. Available at: https://gaia-x.eu/about/

Association (IDSA)[6] to promote the use of data spaces throughout Europe and at other locations [40].

Among the multiple key factors needed for the establishment of European data spaces are the following: intellectual property, legislative instruments, funding programmes, data sharing, and the development of a data workforce. Among the current achievements of the Data Spaces Business Alliance are the development of a "Technical Convergence Discussion Document", a workable document that outlines a single reference technology framework on the basis of the technical convergence of current architectures and models and the shared infrastructure and implementation activities of utilities. The aim of this document, which has already been endorsed by the Data Spaces Support Centre, is to achieve interoperability and portability of solutions across multiple data spaces through the coordinated integration of its technological components, which is a key step for the foundation of effective data spaces in Europe and across the globe [42]. Importantly, some organizations, such as the Big Data Value Association, argue that data spaces act as "enablers" that provide the capacity to unleash the potential of data to the European region.

This position is aligned with the European Commission plan for the development of "made in Europe" AI technologies, which should be the result of "large, secure and robust" datasets that are needed for the development of European AI technology. Wide data availability is also a prerequisite for developing AI that can compete with the AI produced by countries such as the United States or China [43]. However, to support the foundation of data spaces and their utilization in various fields, such as AI, legislative instruments that involve different sectors are needed. In this context, instruments have been proposed or adopted in correspondence with the European strategy for data, including the Regulation (EU) 2022/868 (Data Governance Act), which aims to establish guidance on the use of business data to promote its availability, the Implementing Act on High Value Datasets,[7] and the Regulation (EU) 2023/2854 (Data Act), which aims to establish a ∫ for data to allow data to flow freely within the EU, as well as other legislative instruments related to the use, interpretation, portability, and other aspects of datasets [40], such as the European Health Data Space Regulation, described in the next paragraph.

Another important step in the development of data spaces for the European region, which is already taking place, is the support of these spaces through funding programmes. For this purpose, the European Commission has already developed multiple funding programmes, such as the Digital Europe Programme (DIGITAL), the Horizon Europe programme for research and innovation, the Connecting Europe

---

[6] The International Data Spaces Association (IDSA) is a nonprofit organization dedicated to developing and advocating for standards that enable data spaces—secure environments where organizations can share data while maintaining complete control over how it is used. Available at: https://internationaldataspaces.org/

[7] On 22 December 2022, the European Commission's DG CNECT adopted the long-awaited Implementing Act on a list of High-Value Datasets. This comes as an implementation decision following up the Directive on open data and the reuse of public sector information replaces and enhances the "PSI Directive" (2003/98/EC)

Facility (CEF) for digital infrastructures and other projects, including programmes at the regional level involving multiple countries, which will collaborate to develop the technical infrastructure necessary for the development of data spaces [40]. The goal of the European data strategy is to establish a single data market that guarantees Europe's data sovereignty and global competitiveness. Additionally, the common European data spaces facilitate and promote the use of data in the economy and society, while control of data remains in the hands of those who generate it, whether they are companies, individuals, etc.

As part of the structuring process for this vision to take place, the Data Spaces Support Centre (DSSC) was developed with the mission of creating common data spaces that collectively could develop a sovereign, interoperable, and trustworthy data sharing environment. Additionally, it aims to "enable data reuse within and across sectors, fully respecting EU values, and supporting the European Economy and society" [41] The DSSC has been founded with the vision of exploring the multiple needs of data space initiatives, as well as collaborating in the definition of common requirements and the establishment of best practices to speed up the formation of sovereign data spaces as a fundamental aspect of digital transformation [42]. The successful creation and adoption of a pan-European data sharing platform has the potential to develop into a significant turning point for the development of a new data economy. Moreover, the integration of existing vertical, cross-sectoral, personal, and industrial data spaces could, if integrated into this macro level, not only provide additional services and opportunities for experimentation to all stakeholders but also support the promotion of key identifying characteristics for the European region, such as privacy and equity. This, in part, should be the result of secure, fair, and trustworthy legal, regulatory, and governance frameworks that should take place alongside the development of Pan-European data sharing platforms [43].

Among the opportunities that have shown marked interest for industrial players, national- and European-level legislative institutions, and other stakeholders (and, as such, offer the capacity to promote the integration or creation of job opportunities for the new European data workforce) are as follows: (1) data sharing tools and technologies that are used for the alignment and integration of data; (2) architectures, standards, protocols, and governance models that aim to unlock data silos; (3) business models centred on capitalization of the value of data assets, including those implementing AI technologies; and (4) leveraged initiatives across the Pan-European region that enable data analytics and sharing across the region [43]. Common European data spaces are categorized into nine different spaces, including a health data space, which will play a crucial role in the advancement of healthcare systems, thereby improving areas such as the detection, diagnosis, and treatment of diseases and evidence-based decision-making [44]. A DSSC is composed of 12 consortium partners, combining its expertise to enable the use of multiple tools for the development of data spaces and contributing to the generation of sustainable and scalable products, which could help the global market use shared data for business models or policy making processes [45]. Strategies and investments should also support the development of the European data workforce. Some organizations that play crucial roles in this process are the Big Data Value Public Private Partnership (BDV PPP) and its members, as well as the Big Data Value Association (BDVA).

3.4   Chance of the European Health Data Space Regulation

On 3 May 2022, a legislative proposal aimed at supporting the development of a single EU market for data was presented by the European Commission as a pillar of the European Health Union [46]. In spring 2024, the European Parliament and the Council reached a political agreement on the Commission proposal for the European Health Data Space regulation, which entered into force in spring 2025. Among its goals are the harmonization and standardization of electronic health data exchange within European Union countries to facilitate the delivery of healthcare across borders, as well as the empowerment of individuals regarding access to their personal electronic health data, thereby allowing them to take control of their healthcare process. Furthermore, the regulation aims to provide a consistent, trustworthy, and efficient structure for reusing health data for the public interest, as in the fields of medical research and innovation, health policy making and regulatory activities. To build such an ecosystem, a key aspect of European Health Data Space (EHDS) regulation is the assurance of health data interoperability at the technical, semantical, and organizational levels [47] by creating a shared EU framework that includes infrastructures, governance tools, and rules to support both the primary and secondary uses of electronic health data.

Currently, in many EU countries, natural persons still face challenges in practising rights such as access to and transfer of their personal health data both domestically and internationally. This is in violation of the provisions of Regulation (EU) 2016/679 (hereafter referred to as the "GDPR"), which protects natural persons' rights over their data, including health data. Furthermore, health data regulations in EU Member States reveal inconsistent applications and interpretations of the GDPR by Member States, resulting in significant legal ambiguity [48],[8] which in turn also creates obstacles to the secondary use of electronic health data. The barriers preventing researchers, innovators, regulators, and policy makers from accessing the electronic health data they need consequently create situations in which natural persons cannot benefit from innovative treatments and policy makers cannot effectively respond to a health crisis. Furthermore, producers of digital health goods and suppliers of digital health services operating in one member state encounter barriers and extra expenses when they enter another because of disparate standards and restricted interoperability. The European Health Data Space Regulation seeks to guarantee a safe processing environment and a legal framework made up of reliable EU and Member State governance mechanisms. To improve natural person well-

---

[8] European Commission, Assessment of the EU Member States' rules on health data in the light of the GDPR, 2021

being, diagnosis, and treatment, this would enable researchers, innovators, policy makers, and regulators at the EU and Member State levels to access pertinent electronic health data. This would result in better and more informed policies. Harmonizing regulations also aims to increase the efficiency of the healthcare system by facilitating the emergence of a single market for digital health goods and services [49].

EHDS regulation appears to be innovative legislation despite moving from other previous approaches. The first mention of eHealth in EU law was found in Article 14 of Directive 2011/24/EU on the application of patients' rights in cross-border healthcare (referred to as the "CBHC Directive"). The impact assessment of the EHDS indicates that the applicable CBHC Directive provisions are optional, which may partially explain why this aspect of the Directive has demonstrated very low effectiveness in terms of secondary uses of electronic health data and limited effectiveness in supporting natural persons' control over their personal electronic health data at the national and international levels. The COVID-19 pandemic also confirmed the critical need and great potential for harmonization and interoperability, enhancing national technical expertise already in place. Better access to and exchange of various forms of electronic health data, such as patient registries, genomics data, and electronic health records, was considered a goal of the EHDS regulation, which also promotes several secondary uses (such as research, innovation, policy making, and regulatory purposes) in addition to supporting healthcare delivery. Additionally, it will set up systems for data altruism in the medical field.

EHDS regulation contributed to the realization of the Digital Compass[9] goal of granting 100% of natural persons access to their medical records, the Commission's vision for the EU's digital transformation by 2030, and the Declaration of Digital Principles.[10] The EHDS will also provide support to the European Health Emergency Preparedness and Response Authority (HERA),[11] the European Union Mission on Cancer,[12] the Pharmaceutical Strategy for Europe,[13] and Europe's Beating Cancer Plan,[14] aiming at establishing a technological and legislative framework that facilitates, among other advancements, novel pharmaceuticals, vaccines, medical equipment, and in vitro diagnostics for timely detection, prevention, and treatment of health emergencies. Furthermore, by facilitating safe cross-border access and sharing among healthcare practitioners in the EU, including the exchange of data pertaining to natural persons with cancer, the EHDS regulation contributes to the advancement of knowledge, prevention, early detection, diagnosis, treatment, and monitoring of cancer [49].

---

[9] European Commission, Europe's digital decade: digital trends for 2030
[10] European Commission, Initiative on Declaration of Digital Principles – the European way for the digital society
[11] Health Emergency Preparedness and Response Authority
[12] EU Mission: Cancer | European Commission (europa.eu).
[13] A pharmaceutical strategy for Europe (europa.eu).
[14] A cancer plan for Europe | European Commission (europa.eu).

The framework for the secondary use of electronic health data provided by the EHDS regulation is in line with other relevant EU regulations in the field of data strategy, such as Regulation (EU) 2022/868 (Data Governance Act) and Regulation (EU) 2023/2854 (Data Act). However, EHDS represents an important step forward for the healthcare sector. In fact, the Data Governance Act does not establish a true right to the secondary use of public sector data; rather, it establishes general guidelines for such use according to its horizontal extent. The Data Act, which improves the portability of some user-generated data, which may include health data, does not establish rules for all health data. On the other hand, the EHDS provides more precise rules addressing health data use and governance in the healthcare sector and complements these horizontal legislative acts on data, in general. It is a key milestone not only in promoting cross-border healthcare but also in facilitating medical research and other secondary uses in the public interest, serving as a catalyst for the integration of large health datasets.

The implementation of EHDS regulation requires the participation of multiple stakeholders in a highly complex scenario, implying obligations and opportunities. Data holders and Health Data Access Bodies (HDABs) play the most important role in enabling electronic health data access for secondary purposes once a data applicant (becoming a data user once they are allowed by the access bodies) applies for it. The category of health data holders includes public, not for-profit or private entities that are providers of the health and/or care sectors; providers carrying out research or developing products or services within these sectors, such as hospitals and other healthcare organizations (such as clinics and nursing home ambulatories); professional associations; medical research organizations; pharmaceutical and insurance companies; companies developing wellness applications; and public health institutions. EU institutions, bodies, offices, or agencies that process electronic health data as well as mortality registries are included in the data holder category, whereas natural persons and microenterprises are exempted—except for single Member States that disagree on that—to preserve them from a disproportionate administrative burden.

Data holders make the electronic health data available for data applicants/users on the basis of a data permit or request issued by the Health Data Access Bodies, which allows the processing of health data for secondary purposes, including special categories of data under Article 9(2) of the GDPR. Health Data Access Bodies ensure the need for safeguards (in terms of lawful purposes, trusted governance, and a secure processing environment) for personal electronic health data processing for secondary use. The EU Member States do not need to maintain or introduce further conditions under Article 9(4) of the GDPR, including limitations and specific provisions requesting the consent of natural persons. However, they can introduce measures and additional safeguards at the national level aimed at safeguarding the sensitivity and value of certain categories of data. The Health Data Access Bodies assess the information provided by health data applicants to check if it fulfils the requirements and conditions set out in EHDS regulations before releasing a data permit for the processing of personal electronic health data held by health data holders.

To comply with their role and functions as required by the EHDS regulation, HDABs must build digital business capabilities. These include some essentials that are mandatory and reported below.

1. **The health dataset catalogue** enables data applicants/users to find datasets, thus facilitating health data discoverability for secondary uses (this capability includes the publication of accurate and regularly updated health dataset descriptions and labels regarding data quality and utility).
2. **The data access application and management system** enable the assessment of the data access applications and of the data requests by a data applicant/data user,[15] from receiving a data access application to providing an outcome for that data access application. This is the system used to manage applications and to manage the decision about the applications in three months with the help of an application evaluation committee. The user can also ask for an update or an amendment of its data access application, which is managed by the data access application and management system.
3. **The permit issuing** releases the permit, allowing access to those applications that have received a positive decision. Unlike the data access application management system, permit issuing concerns the release of a permit, which is a contract between the HDAB and the data user establishing the conditions for the requested access, including the fees to pay and the duration of the access. The HDAB can revoke an issued permit if the data user makes something that is not compliant with the EHDS regulation. Once the permit is revoked, the data user cannot continue to access the data.
4. **The secure processing environment (SPE)** allows data use according to the permit that was issued (see point 3). Each HDAB needs to configure the secure processing environment enabling specific data access (who has access, what data must be there, for how long the secure processing environment is open for access, and how the requested dataset is brought into the secure processing environment). In the processing environment, the data user analyses the datasets: the possible processing operations are defined in the permit, eventually including the data user bringing algorithms to run over the data. Finally, the data user extracts the results, which are not personal information.
5. **The cross-border gateway** enables the connection of HDABs with the HealthData@EU platform[16] for several functions, such as sharing national dataset descriptions with the EU dataset catalogue, receiving data access applica-

---

[15] The output of a data access application followed by a data permit is the access to anonymized or pseudonymized dataset in a secure processing environment, while the output of a data request is the access to aggregated data in a statistical form.

[16] The HealthData@EU Central Platform is a pivotal digital system being developed by the European Commission to meet the requirements of the European Health Data Space regulation. This platform hosts the EU Dataset Catalogue, which compiles metadata from member states, European institutions, third countries, and research infrastructures. The HealthData@EU infrastructure is the machine-to-machine connection (based on the eDelivery AS4 software infrastructure) between the Central Platform and the contact points for secondary use at the national level.

tions from EU Central Services, and sharing SPE descriptions with the EU SPE list. For example, the data access application management system at the HDAB level needs to be able to receive through the cross-border gateway an application that comes from the EU portal [50].

6. **The transparency portal**, which publishes decisions regarding data access applications or data requests, publishes penalties regarding data users or data holders when they do not fulfil their obligations, publishes results from projects on secondary uses realized through the secure processing environment and the HealthData@EU infrastructure, and publishes the opt-out procedure, which must be publicly explained to allow people to exercise the right to opt out. The publication of the opt-out procedure in the transparency portal is thus related to another capability for HDABs, which is the opt-out management capability to enable the natural person to exercise the right to opt out.

7. **The system can manage supervision, monitoring, compliance, and penalties** for data holders or data users, enabling functionalities related to tracking, documenting, and being aware of these activities.

There are other capabilities that could be implemented to sustain those that are mandatory for HDABs according to the EHDS regulation. For example, to allow an efficient publication of health dataset descriptions by HDABs, these entities should be strictly connected with all the health data holders that provide datasets and their descriptions. For this reason, the creation within the HDABs of a Data Holder Space as a nonmandatory but highly relevant business capability could facilitate the implementation of the health dataset catalogue (which is mandatory), especially in the cases of complex data holders such as cross-border registries, trusted data holders,[17] and intermediate entities. Key functionalities of a Data Holder Space include an accreditation system of the data holders and a management centre to track and trace the information regarding data holders accredited in each Member State (listing them in a registry), which are obliged to provide dataset descriptions and data quality and utility labels through a communication system that can be personalized by each Member State.

The interactions with data users can also benefit from a capability (a Data User Space) dedicated to satisfying the need of HDABs for additional information or clarifications from a data applicant/user to comply with obligations and/or to manage the payment of fees by the data applicant/user, monitoring and tracking in the conversations with the data users and the time missing for the 3-month deadline established by the EHDS regulation to complete the data application assessment.

---

[17] Trusted data holders are those which have particularly advanced and reliable experience in the digital business capabilities that are required to the HDABs by the EHDS regulation (e.g. data access application assessment, secure processing environment in which the data user can access to the data) and already created the enabling conditions in their work environment. For this reason, they can support the HDABs in their capabilities acting on behalf of them. Consequently, trusted data holders have more responsibilities than simple data holders which have only two obligations: (1) provide the health dataset description and set; (2) make health data available when the HDAB requests those data.

The data user can be authenticated through the It is the responsibility of each country to implement their e-IDAS node provider,[18] which is the central identity provider at the EU level [51].

To provide to a data applicant/user an answer regarding a data access application, the HDAB capabilities could also include a nonmandatory but relevant setting dedicated to access application evaluation, including, for example, a fee management system that sets fees, issues invoices, and allows data users to pay fees, compensating HDABs for the amount of time that is going to be spent evaluating the data application form that data applicant/user. Therefore, this capability would be useful for setting the fee and creating a way for the data user to pay that fee.

EU Member States have started to establish Health Data Access Bodies as competent authorities responsible for the secondary use of health data under the EHDS framework, either *ex novo* or by adapting existing national bodies capable of carrying out their functions. A Community of Practice of Health Data Access Bodies for secondary use (EHDS2 Community of Practice) has also been established by EU Member States with the support of the European Commission [52]. This community facilitates the interaction between Health Data Access Bodies from different EU Member States through a common platform enabling the sharing of best practices, challenges, and concerns, as well as the strengthening of collaborations to build and manage their tasks. The community also aims to ensure a common understanding of the EHDS Regulation in the field of secondary use and to enable a continuous exchange of information on national laws, plans, and strategies for a harmonized implementation of the EHDS in the EU. On the basis of common technical specifications and procedures in the field of secondary use, the EHDS2 Community is working at building the necessary business capacities of HDABs.

The EHDS2 Community is composed of a general assembly, a steering committee, six thematic working subgroups that guide the Member States in the definition, implementation, and operation of the Health Data Access Bodies, on the basis of the provisions of the EHDS Regulation as the health data access application, the catalogues of metadata and the quality of health datasets, the secure environments for the processing of health data, and the cross-border gateways. It also includes horizontal thematic working subgroups focused on the coordination of operational aspects and the stakeholders' fora.

---

[18] The eIDAS-Network consists of a number of interconnected eIDAS-Nodes, one per participating country, which can either request or provide cross-border authentication. It is the responsibility of each country to implement their eIDAS-Node and support the connection of national Identity Providers and Attribute Providers to the eIDAS-Node, thus making their national eID schemes accessible to cross-border online services.

The European Commission through the DIGITAL programme provides this tool for anyone to display the current interconnections between the eIDAS-Nodes of the eIDAS-Network based on the declaration by the Member States.

References

1. World Health Organization (2023) Monitoring the implementation of digital health: an over-view of selected national and international methodologies. https://www.who.int/europe/news-room/events/item/2023/02/16/default-calendar/monitoring-the-implementation-of-digital-health%2D%2Dan-overview-of-selected-national-and-international-methodologies. Accessed 28 Dec 2023
2. World Health Organization (WHO) (2022) Monitoring the implementation of digital health: an overview of selected national and international methodologies. https://www.who.int/europe/publications/i/item/WHO-EURO-2022-5985-45750-65816. Accessed 29 Jun 2024
3. Liaw ST, Zhou R, Ansari S, Gao J (2021) A digital health profile & maturity assessment tool-kit: cocreation and testing in the Pacific Islands. J Am Med Inform Assoc 28:494–503. https://doi.org/10.1093/JAMIA/OCAA255
4. Burmann A, Meister S (2021) Practical application of maturity models in healthcare: findings from multiple digitalization case studies. In: Pesquita C, Fred AH (eds) Proceedings of the 14th International Joint Conference on Biomedical Engineering Systems and Technologies, Volume 5: HEALTHINF. SciTePress, Setúbal, pp 100–110
5. Doctor E, Eymann T, Fürstenau D et al (2023) A maturity model for assessing the digitaliza-tion of public health agencies: development and evaluation. Bus Inf Syst Eng 65:539–554. https://doi.org/10.1007/S12599-023-00813-Y/TABLES/3
6. NHS England (2023) Digital maturity assessment. https://www.england.nhs.uk/digitaltechnol-ogy/connecteddigitalsystems/digital-maturity-assessment/. Accessed 29 Jun 2024
7. Arora A, Wright A, Cheng M et al (2021) Innovation pathways in the NHS: an introductory review. Ther Innov Regul Sci 55:1045–1058. https://doi.org/10.1007/S43441-021-00304-W
8. Johnston DS (2017) Digital maturity: are we ready to use technology in the NHS? Future Healthc J 4:189–192. https://doi.org/10.7861/FUTUREHOSP.4-3-189
9. Cresswell K, Sheikh A, Krasuska M et al (2019) Reconceptualizing the digital maturity of health systems. Lancet Digit Health 1:e200–e201. https://doi.org/10.1016/S2589-7500(19)30083-4
10. Snowdon A, Hussein A, Olubisi A, Wright A (2024) Digital maturity as a strategy for advanc-ing patient experience in US hospitals. J Patient Exp 11:23743735241228932. https://doi.org/10.1177/23743735241228931
11. Teixeira F, Li E, Laranjo L et al (2023) Digital maturity and its determinants in general practice: a cross-sectional study in 20 countries. Front Public Health 10:962924. https://doi.org/10.3389/FPUBH.2022.962924/BIBTEX
12. American Hospital Association (2020) Leveraging data for health care innovation. Maturity framework: data-driven health care organization
13. EY Sweden (2023) Nordic care model: challenges, opportunities and the future. https://www.ey.com/en_se/health-sciences-wellness/nordic-care-model-challenges-opportunities-and-future. Accessed 29 Jun 2024
14. Ernst & Young LLP (2023) Shaping the next generation of digital and data-driven healthcare and sustainable practices. https://assets.ey.com/content/dam/ey-sites/ey-com/en_in/topics/esg/04/ey-pharma-sustainability-esg-perspectives.pdf. Accessed 28 Dec 2023
15. Bi WL, Hosny A, Schabath MB et al (2019) Artificial intelligence in cancer imaging: clini-cal challenges and applications. CA Cancer J Clin 69:127–157. https://doi.org/10.3322/CAAC.21552
16. Kamdar JH, Praba JJ, Georrge JJ (2020) Artificial intelligence in medical diagnosis: methods, algorithms and applications. In: Jain V, Chatterjee JM (eds) Machine learning with health care perspective. Learning and analytics in intelligent systems, vol 13. Springer, Cham, pp 27–37
17. The Swedish National Council on Medical Ethics (Smer) (2020) In brief – Artificial intel-ligence in healthcare. https://smer.se/en/2020/05/28/in-brief-artificial-intelligence-in-healthcare/. Accessed 28 Dec 2023

18. Cossy-Gantner A, Germann S, Schwalbe NR, Wahl B (2018) Artificial intelligence (AI) and global health: how can AI contribute to health in resource-poor settings? BMJ Glob Health 3:e000798. https://doi.org/10.1136/BMJGH-2018-000798

19. Tang X (2020) The role of artificial intelligence in medical imaging research. BJR Open 2:20190031. https://doi.org/10.1259/BJRO.20190031

20. Pinto-Coelho L (2023) How artificial intelligence is shaping medical imaging technology: a survey of innovations and applications. Bioengineering 10:1435. https://doi.org/10.3390/BIOENGINEERING10121435

21. Schwalbe N, Wahl B (2020) Artificial intelligence and the future of global health. Lancet 395:1579–1586. https://doi.org/10.1016/S0140-6736(20)30226-9

22. Whitelaw S, Mamas MA, Topol E, Van Spall HGC (2020) Applications of digital technology in COVID-19 pandemic planning and response. Lancet Digit Health 2:e435–e440. https://doi.org/10.1016/S2589-7500(20)30142-4

23. Privacy International (2021) Microtargeting. https://privacyinternational.org/learn/microtargeting. Accessed 28 Dec 2023

24. NBC News, Harris B (2021) As vaccine demand slows, doctors shift to "microtargeting" vulnerable communities. https://www.nbcnews.com/news/us-news/vaccine-demand-slows-doctors-shift-microtargeting-vulnerable-communities-n1266031. Accessed 28 Dec 2023

25. CDC Foundation (2023) What is public health? https://www.cdcfoundation.org/what-public-health. Accessed 28 Dec 2023

26. Russell S, Norvig P (2021) Artificial intelligence: a modern approach, 4th edn. Pearson, London

27. Morgenstern JD, Rosella LC, Daley MJ et al (2021) "AI's gonna have an impact on everything in society, so it has to have an impact on public health": a fundamental qualitative descriptive study of the implications of artificial intelligence for public health. BMC Public Health 21:40. https://doi.org/10.1186/S12889-020-10030-X

28. Alcantara MF, Cao Y, Liu C et al (2017) Improving tuberculosis diagnostics using deep learning and mobile health technologies among resource-poor communities in Perú. Smart Health 1–2:66–76. https://doi.org/10.1016/J.SMHL.2017.04.003

29. Roski J, Hamilton BA, Chapman W et al (2019) How artificial intelligence is changing health and health care. In: Matheny M, Israni ST, Whicher D, Ahmed M (eds) Artificial intelligence in health care: the hope, the hype, the promise, the Peril. National Academies Press, Washington, DC, pp 65–98

30. Bourguet JR, Thomopoulos R, Mugnier ML, Abécassis J (2013) An artificial intelligence-based approach to deal with argumentation applied to food quality in a public health policy. Expert Syst Appl 40:4539–4546. https://doi.org/10.1016/J.ESWA.2013.01.059

31. Larburu N, Artetxe A, Escolar V et al (2018) Artificial intelligence to prevent mobile heart failure patients decompensation in real time: monitoring-based predictive model. Mob Inf Syst 2018:1546210. https://doi.org/10.1155/2018/1546210

32. Lakhani CM, Tierney BT, Manrai AK et al (2019) Repurposing large health insurance claims data to estimate genetic and environmental contributions in 560 phenotypes. Nat Genet 51:327–334. https://doi.org/10.1038/S41588-018-0313-7

33. Khemasuwan D, Sorensen JS, Colt HG (2020) Artificial intelligence in pulmonary medicine: computer vision, predictive model and COVID-19. Eur Respir Rev 29:200181. https://doi.org/10.1183/16000617.0181-2020

34. Patel CJ, Rasooly D, Khoury MJ (2019) Data science and machine learning in public health: promises and challenges. https://blogs.cdc.gov/genomics/2019/09/20/data-science/. Accessed 28 Dec 2023

35. Topol EJ (2019) High-performance medicine: the convergence of human and artificial intelligence. Nat Med 25:44–56. https://doi.org/10.1038/S41591-018-0300-7

36. Hibbard JH, Greene J (2013) What the evidence shows about patient activation: better health outcomes and care experiences; fewer data on costs. Health Aff (Millwood) 32:207–214. https://doi.org/10.1377/HLTHAFF.2012.1061

37. Bu F, Fancourt D (2021) How is patient activation related to healthcare service utilization? Evidence from electronic patient records in England. BMC Health Serv Res 21:1196. https://doi.org/10.1186/S12913-021-07115-7
38. Raj M, de Vries R, Nong P et al (2020) Do people have an ethical obligation to share their health information? Comparing narratives of altruism and health information sharing in a nationally representative sample. PLoS One 15:e0244767. https://doi.org/10.1371/JOURNAL.PONE.0244767
39. Jones RD, Krenz C, Griffith KA et al (2021) Patient experiences, trust, and preferences for health data sharing. JCO Oncol Pract 18:e339–e350. https://doi.org/10.1200/OP.21.00491
40. Eimear F, Marco M, Alexander K et al (2023) European data spaces - scientific insights into data sharing and utilization at scale. Publications Office of the European Union, Luxembourg
41. Data Spaces Support Centre (2023) Mission and vision. https://dssc.eu/space/Mission/175308804/Mission+and+Vision. Accessed 29 Jun 2024
42. Data Spaces Support Centre (2023) Achieving convergence in data spaces. https://dssc.eu/space/News/blog/247037960/DSSC+Insight+Series%3A+Achieving+convergence+in+data+spaces. Accessed 29 Dec 2023
43. Big Data Value Association (2019) Towards a European Data sharing space: enabling data exchange and unlocking AI potential. https://www.bdva.eu/towards-european-data-sharing-space-bdva-position-paper. Accessed 29 Dec 2023
44. Real-time Linked Dataspaces (2023) Common European data spaces. https://dataspaces.info/common-european-data-spaces/#page-content. Accessed 29 Dec 2023
45. Data Spaces Support Centre (2023) Data Spaces Support Centre. https://dssc.eu/. Accessed 29 Dec 2023
46. European Commission (2024) European Health Union. https://commission.europa.eu/strategy-and-policy/priorities-2019-2024/promoting-our-european-way-life/european-health-union_en. Accessed 9 Jan 2025
47. Stellmach C, Muzoora MR, Thun S (2022) Digitalization of health data: interoperability of the proposed European health data space. Stud Health Technol Inform 298:132–136. https://doi.org/10.3233/SHTI220922
48. European Commission (2021) Assessment of the EU member states' rules on health data in the light of GDPR. https://health.ec.europa.eu/system/files/2021-02/ms_rules_health-data_en_0.pdf. Accessed 29 Jun 2024
49. European Commission, Directorate-General for Health and Food Safety (2022) Proposal for a regulation of the European Parliament and of the Council on the European health data space. COM, p 197. https://eur-lex.europa.eu/legal-content/EN/TXT/?uri=CELEX%3A52022PC0197. Accessed 23 Nov 2023
50. European Union (2024) HealthData@EU. https://acceptance.data.health.europa.eu/. Accessed 9 Jan 2025
51. European Commission (2024) eIDAS dashboard. https://eidas.ec.europa.eu/efda/browse/notification/eid-chapter-contacts/IT. Accessed 9 Jan 2025
52. European Commission (2024) Health data access bodies – community of practice. https://health.ec.europa.eu/ehealth-digital-health-and-care/eu-cooperation/health-data-access-bodies-community-practice_en. Accessed 9 Jan 2025

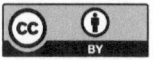

Index